Functional Analytic Psychotherapy

Creating Intense and
Curative Therapeutic Relationships

Functional Analytic Psychotherapy

Creating Intense and
Curative Therapeutic Relationships

Robert J. Kohlenberg
University of Washington
Seattle, Washington

and

Mavis Tsai
Clinical Psychologist in Private Practice
Seattle, Washington

PLENUM PRESS • NEW YORK AND LONDON

Library of Congress Cataloging-in-Publication Data

Kohlenberg, Robert J.
   Functional analytic psychotherapy : creating intense and
curative therapeutic relationships / Robert J. Kohlenberg and Mavis
Tsai.
      p.   cm.
   Includes bibliographical references and index.
   ISBN 0-306-43857-7
   1. Behavior therapy. 2. Psychotherapist and patient. I. Tsai,
Mavis. II. Title.
   [DNLM: 1. Behavior. 2. Professional-Patient Relations.
3. Psychoanalytic Therapy. WM 460.6 K79f]
RC489.B4K65 1991
616.89'142--dc20
DNLM/DLC
for Library of Congress   91-21357
                                                    CIP

10 9 8 7 6 5 4 3 2

ISBN 0-306-43857-7

© 1991 Plenum Press, New York
A Division of Plenum Publishing Corporation
233 Spring Street, New York, N.Y. 10013

Printed in the United States of America

To our parents,
Jack and Bess Kohlenberg
Edwin and Emily Tsai,
whose steadfast love, support, and pride
provided the foundation
for our strivings and accomplishments.

Preface

This book was born out of the many years of collective experience in treating and thinking about our clients. We view this work as a treatment manual with guidelines for creating deep, intense, meaningful, and healing therapeutic relationships. It is not a collection of techniques, although a fair share of them are included. Instead, we have described a conceptual framework that is intended to guide a therapist's activity. Although the theory we use is particularly well suited for this purpose, as soon as we name it, we lose most of our audience. Thus, our desire to impart intellectual stimulation and to share our clinical insights is hampered by the very vehicle on which we rely.

Clinicians do not easily take on new techniques that are given to them in a book. They are particularly unlikely to be receptive if the theory on which these techniques are based causes a strong, negative reaction. This theory, however, is widely misinterpreted and misunderstood; as a consequence, the first chapter contains explanations of the major tenets of radical behaviorism and addresses some of these misunderstandings (You may not have noticed, but we slipped in the name of the theory.) In Chapter 1, we also show how radical behaviorism leads to a focus on the client-therapist relationship.

This book was intended to be read more or less in sequence, but it does not have to be. Each chapter can almost stand alone because many of the lesser known concepts are reviewed, even though they may have appeared in an earlier chapter. The more theoretical and abstract writings occur in the first three chapters, and greater emphasis is placed on clinical application in the chapters that follow. For some, reading the more clinical chapters first might pique interest in perusing the earlier theoretical chapters. We hope that as you go through the chapters and observe how the concepts are applied in new ways, there will be a cumulative effect and the concepts will become more understandable.

In the second chapter, we lay out the principles of doing functional analytic psychotherapy (FAP). Although we provide five principles, only the first one is really needed, and we hope it will be the one you will remember: it is "watch for clinically relevant behaviors"; that is what this book is all about.

Perhaps the third chapter might prove to be the most difficult. It is the first time that some of the concepts of verbal behavior are introduced. A system for analyzing what clients say is explained. An "escape hatch" is provided for those readers who do not wish to spend time in learning the system and who wish to proceed directly to its major conclusions.

Emotions and affect are central to the therapeutic process. We have followed a slightly different road, however, from most other therapeutic systems. Our conclusions are that, on the one hand, feelings do not cause a client's problems, nor are they responsible for therapeutic change. But, on the other hand, therapy cannot work if feelings do not occur. This paradox and others are explained in Chapter 4, where, it is hoped, our discussion on expressing feelings brings additional clarity to this confusing topic.

Everybody thinks and has cognitions. Not only that, but cognitions can play a major role in therapy. In Chapter 5, we give the radical behavioral view of these phenomena in a new way. The result is an approach that we think will be useful to psychotherapists, including cognitive therapists.

In this book, we have extended the application of behavioral theory beyond its usual domain. This extension occurs in its greatest degree in Chapter 6, which deals with problems of the self, a topic not usually discussed in behavioral circles. We present the self as a highly personal experience that comes in many forms, some more adaptive than others. Among the maladaptive forms that we discuss are borderline, narcissistic, and multiple personality disorders. We explain self problems as the result of various external conditions that take place during normal and pathological childhood development.

In Chapter 7, we challenge the contention that the FAP focus on the therapeutic relationship is simply psychoanalysis revisited. The psychoanalytic concepts of transference and therapeutic alliance, and the relational model of object relations therapy, are examined, and a case is made for how FAP occupies a unique niche between psychodynamic and current behavior therapies.

Depending on their interests, readers may think that we saved the best for last. Our final chapter delves into ethical precautions, the supervisory process, the problems inherent in traditional research methodology and its implications for FAP research, and how the principles of FAP can be extended to address problems in the world outside of therapy.

A word needs to be said about the behavioral terminology used throughout the book. Behavioral language helps to give new insights into clinical phenomena and conveys what we are trying to say about how therapy helps and why clients have the problems they do. This terminology was not developed in the psychotherapy environment, however, and is thus cumbersome when used to communicate about phenomena that occur there. We walked a line between the language of radical behaviorists and that used by most clinicians. Sometimes we went north and sometimes south, but we tried to capitalize on the richness of both.

This book emerged from a chapter that originally appeared in Neil Jacobson's edited volume *Psychotherapists in Clinical Practice* (1987). We are grateful to Neil for encouraging us to take that first step. In the present volume, we have facilitated clinical application by giving more attention to client verbal behavior and by using case transcripts. The chapter on the self evolved from a paper originally written by Robert Kohlenberg and Marsha Linehan.

Bob Kohlenberg wishes to acknowledge the importance of his daughter Barbara in the genesis of this book, as she was responsible for reigniting a burned-out radical behaviorist. His son Andy contributed an important perspective on ethics, whereas his son Paul reminded him of the significance of a curious mind, good humor, and commitment. His brother David was always there to listen, which was essential to the completion of this book. His precious co-author, Mavis, infused his life with her limitless love and intellect, which provided the threads that are the core of FAP.

Mavis Tsai cherishes the memory of Ned Wagner, her first graduate advisor. His enthusiasm about her ideas and writings when she was a neophyte graduate student was a priceless gift. In two short years, Ned instilled in her lifetimes of confidence, curiosity, and compassion. Her two other graduate advisors, Stanley Sue and Shirley Feldman-Summers, also played essential and greatly valued roles in her development as a psychologist. Other mentors include Laura Brown, James Coleman, and Ron Smith. Bob, her co-author and partner in life, has enriched the meaning and joy of her life beyond measure with his passionate love, fertile mind, and wondrous presence.

Fellow clinicians Carla Bradshaw, Barbara Johnstone, Karen Lindner, Vickie Sears, Ellen Sherwood, and Alejandra Suarez read part or all of the manuscript in progress and provided important feedback.

We are especially indebted to Anne Uemura, a friend and colleague of the highest order, who spent countless hours poring over every word of our manuscript and giving us detailed and constructive criticism.

The late Willard Day was a great inspiration. His work showed that interpretation is an essential activity of the radical behaviorist. His delight for fledgling ideas provided a haven in which they could grow and flourish.

Steve Hayes paved the way in applying radical behavioral principles to adult psychotherapy. Stanley Messer, the first psychodynamically oriented scholar who took our work seriously, gave us invaluable critical feedback.

To the next generation of FAP therapists—Michael Addis, James Cordova, Darla Broberg, Victoria Follette, Allan Fruzzeti, Enrico Ganaulti, Kelly Koerner, Marty Stern, Julian Somers, Paula Truax, and Jennifer Waltz—we thank you all for the give-and-take that occurred while ideas were new and a system was developing.

✓ We are grateful to our clients who have shared with us their deepest pains and joys. Each and every one of our clients has contributed to our clinical acumen and has shaped who we are as therapists. To protect the confidentiality of the clients who are described in the case histories, all names and other identifying information have been changed.

The passing of B. F. Skinner is a great loss to those of us who admired him. The essence of his lifelong work was the hope it offered that we could improve our lives and the world in which we live. We wrote this book in the spirit of that legacy, and regret that he did not get a chance to read it and to see one more of the countless effects his work has had on others.

R.J.K.
M.T.

Contents

Chapter 1

Introduction   1

Philosophical Tenets of Radical Behaviorism   3
   Contextual Nature of Knowledge and Reality   3
   Nonmentalistic View of Behavior: The Focus on
      Environmental Variables That Control Behavior   5
   Focal Interest in Verbal Behavior Controlled by
      Directly Observed Events   6
Theoretical Underpinnings of FAP   7
   Reinforcement   8
   Specification of Clinically Relevant Behavior 13
   Arranging for Generalization 13

Chapter 2

**Clinical Application of Functional Analytic
Psychotherapy** 17

Client Problems and Clinically Relevant Behaviors 17
   CRB1: Client Problems That Occur in Session 18
   CRB2: Client Improvements That Occur in Session 19
   CRB3: Client Interpretations of Behavior 22
   Assessment 23
Therapeutic Technique—The Five Rules 24
   Rule 1: Watch for CRBs 24

Rule 2: Evoke CRBs   26
Rule 3: Reinforce CRB2s   29
Rule 4: Observe the Potentially Reinforcing Effects of
    Therapist Behavior in Relation to Client CRBs   36
Rule 5: Give Interpretations of Variables That Affect
    Client Behavior   37
Case Illustration   42

Chapter 3
Supplementation: Enhancing Therapist Awareness of
Clinically Relevant Behavior   47

Classification of Verbal Behavior   47
    The FAP Client Response Classification System   50
    Classification and the Observation of Clinically
        Relevant Behavior   60
    Examples of Classifications of Client Responses   61
Therapeutic Situations That Frequently Evoke Clinically
    Relevant Behavior   63

Chapter 4
The Role of Emotions and Memories in Behavior
Change   69

Emotions   69
    Learning the Meanings of Feelings   72
    Feelings as Causes of Behavior   73
    Expressing Feelings   75
    Avoiding Feelings   77
    Degree of Contact with Controlling Variables   78
Memories   81
Clinical Implications   84
    Offer a Behavioral Rationale for Getting in Touch with
        Feelings   85
    Increase Private Control of Feelings   86
    Increase Therapist Expression of Feelings   87
    Enhance Client Contact with Controlling Variables   88
Case Illustration   94

Chapter 5
Cognitions and Beliefs   97

Cognitive Therapy   98
    Problems with Cognitive Therapy and the *ABC*
        Paradigm   98
    Revised Formulation of Cognitive Therapy   101
The FAP Revision of $A \rightarrow B \rightarrow C$ 103
    Contingency-Shaped Behavior   104
    Tacts and Mands: Two Types of Verbal Behavior   105
    Rule-Governed Behavior   111
    Cognitive Structures and Contingency-Shaped Behavior . . .   113
Clinical Implications of the FAP View of Beliefs   114
    Focus on Thinking in the Here and Now   114
    Take into Account the Varying Role That Thoughts
        Can Play   116
    Offer Relevant Explanations of Client Problems   119
    Use Direct Cognitive Manipulation with Caution   120
Case Illustration   122

Chapter 6
The Self   125

Common Definitions of the Self   126
A Behavioral Formulation of Self   127
    Basic Concepts   128
    The Emergence of "I" as a Small Functional Unit   132
    Qualities of the "I"   139
Maladaptive Development of the Self Experience   141
    Less Severe Disturbances of the Self   142
    Severe Disturbances of the Self   148
Clinical Implications   157
    Reinforce Talking in the Absence of Specific External
        Cues   158
    Match Therapeutic Tasks to the Level of Private
        Control in the Client's Repertoire   159
    Reinforce as Many Client "I X" Statements as Possible . . .   165

Chapter 7
**Functional Analytic Psychotherapy: A Bridge between
Psychoanalysis and Behavior Therapy**   169

FAP in Contrast with Psychodynamic Approaches   170
    Transference   170
    The Therapeutic Alliance   177
    Object Relations   179
FAP in Contrast with Current Behavior Therapies   182
FAP: A Unique Niche between Psychoanalysis and
    Behavior Therapy   185

Chapter 8
**Reflections on Ethical, Supervisory, Research, and
Cultural Issues**   189

Ethical Issues   189
    Proceed Cautiously   190
    Avoid Sexual Exploitation   191
    Guard against the Continuation of a Nonbeneficial
        Treatment   191
    Be Aware of Prejudicial and Oppressive Values   192
    Avoid Emotional Tyranny   193
FAP Supervision   194
Research and Evaluation   196
    Pitfalls of Traditional Research Paradigms   197
    Alternative Methods of Data Collection that Influence
        Clinical Practice   199
Cultural Problems Due to Loss of Contact   203
Conclusion   207

References   209

Index   215

1

Introduction

> If I look back on those patients whom I have seen change a great deal, I know the heat was in the therapeutic relationship. . . . There was struggle and fear and closeness and love and terror. There was intimacy and outrage, concern and humiliation. . . . It was a journey of importance, more to the patient who had come seeking help, but in fact to both participants. It was a process which carried on throughout the course of therapy and left both patient and therapist altered by the experience. . . The therapeutic relationship is at the absolute heart of psychotherapy, and is the vehicle whereby therapeutic change occurs. (Greben, 1981, pp. 453-454)

Most experienced clinicians, regardless of theoretical orientation, have had memorable clients who changed markedly in ways that far exceeded the stated goals of the therapy. For those clients, Greben's description seems to capture an aspect of what the therapeutic process was like, even if the treatment were based on a theory that is quite different from his psychodynamic perspective. What is missing, however, from Greben's writing and from most systems of therapy that focus on the relationship between therapist and client is a coherent conceptual system with well-defined theoretical constructs that lead to step-by-step therapy guidelines.

We will describe a treatment that has a clear and concise conceptual framework and yet seems to produce what Greben describes. We call our treatment *functional analytic psychotherapy* (FAP), and it is derived, perhaps unexpectedly, from a Skinnerian functional analysis of the typical pyschotherapy environment. Its foundations are in radical behaviorism, the conceptual framework described in the writings of B. F. Skinner (e.g., 1945, 1953, 1957, 1974). The major philosophical tenets of radical behavioral are reviewed in the section that follows.

Although FAP is a type of behavior therapy, it is quite different from traditional behavior therapies, such as social skills training, cognitive restructuring, desensitization, and sex therapy. Instead, FAP techniques are concordant with the expectations of clients who seek an intensive, emotional, in-depth therapy experience. Moreover, it is also well suited for clients who have not improved adequately with traditional behavior therapies, who have difficulties in establishing intimate relationships, and/or who have diffuse, pervasive, interpersonal problems typified by Axis II diagnoses in the DSM-III-R (American Psychiatric Association, 1987). In order to deal with these in-depth problems, FAP leads the therapist into a caring, genuine, sensitive, involving, and emotional relationship with his or her client while at the same time capitalizing on the clarity, logic, and precise definitions of radical behaviorism.

Unfortunately, radical behaviorism has been widely misunderstood and rejected. When we asked our colleagues what came to mind in response to the term *radical behaviorism*, their responses included: (1) "I think about Skinner boxes. I have a visceral sense of rejection. I think it's simplistic, and it denies the reality of a rich complex inner psyche that interacts with external reality. Behaviorism has always seemed very arrogant to me, in the sense that the incredible mystery of being has been reduced to what can be observed" and (2) "Did you hear about the two radical behaviorists who made passionate love? Afterward, one said to the other, 'that was good for you, how was it for me?'" These reactions—that radical behaviorism is simplistic, reduces meaningful behavior down to only that which can be observed, and requires public agreement—are representative of the misunderstandings that most clinicians hold. These distortions are due in part to the esoteric nature of Skinner's writings, which make it hard for him to be interpreted correctly, and also due to the fact that radical behaviorism is often confused with the more widely known methodological or conventional behaviorism. In contrast to radical behaviorism, methodological behaviorism requires public agreement for observations. It thus excludes the direct study of consciousness, feelings, and thinking by focusing only on what is publicly observable. Early on, Skinner (1945) differentiated his approach from the rest of psychology by declaring that his "toothache is just as physical as my typewriter" (p. 294) and rejected the requirement of public agreement. To be accurate, the above joke told by our colleague should start with "Did you hear about the two methodological behaviorists?"

PHILOSOPHICAL TENETS OF RADICAL BEHAVIORISM

When one speaks of "radical," an image of a wild-eyed extremist often comes to mind. It is not generally known that the word *radical* comes from the Latin *radix*, meaning "root." "The proper radical is one who tries to get to the root of things, not to be distracted by superficials, to see the woods for the trees. It is good to be a radical. Anyone who thinks *deeply* will be one" (Peck, 1987, p. 25). Thus, radical behaviorism is a rich and deep theory that tries to get to the root of human behavior. Slips of the tongue, the unconscious, poetry, spirituality, and metaphor are a sampling of subjects that have been discussed by radical behaviorists. Feelings and other private experience are also reckoned with, and "stimulation arising inside the body plays an important part in behavior" (Skinner, 1974, p. 241). Although it is difficult to distill the volumes of Skinner's writings into a brief summary of radical behaviorism, the text that follows is an attempt to describe its basic philosophical tenets.

Contextual Nature of Knowledge and Reality

Skinner rejects the idea that in knowing about something the expression of our knowledge consists of a statement of what the object of knowledge *is*, that it has a more or less permanent identity as a real element of nature. We may attribute "thingness" to events largely because we are accustomed to talking about the world as composed of objects that are felt to possess an inherent constancy or stability. In fact, the discovery of objective truths—the original goal of science—increasingly has been revealed to be untenable. Science at its core is either the behavior of scientists or the artifacts of such activity, and scientific behavior is in turn presumably controlled by the same kind of variables that govern any other aspect of complex human behavior. Thus, scientists are themselves no more than behaving organisms, and the interests and activities of the scientific observer cannot be fully disentangled from the observations that are produced.

This anti-ontological position of Skinner's is similar to a constructivist or Kantian viewpoint (Efran, Lukens & Lukens, 1988). In the eighteenth century, philosopher Immanuel Kant, one of the pillars of Western intellectual tradition, proposed that knowledge is the invention of an active organism interacting with an environment. In contrast, John Locke, founder of British empiricism, saw knowledge as the result of the outside world etching a copy of itself onto initially "blank" minds. Thus, the

Lockean regards mental images as basically "representations" or "discoveries" of something *outside* the organism, whereas the Kantian assumes that mental images are wholly creations or "inventions" of the organism, produced as a by-product of its navigation through life. Constructivists acknowledge the active role they play in creating a view of the world and interpreting observations in terms of it.

Translating these positions in terms of clinical practice, an objectivist enterprise, such as classical psychoanalysis, is built around the belief that objective truth is discoverable, and when properly revealed, leads to improved psychological health. In contrast, the constructivist belief is that a good intervention generates its own truths. Objectivist therapists want to know what really happened in the past; constructivist therapists are more interested in "history" as a key to the unfolding narrative that gives contemporary events their meaning; that is, the history and background of the perceiver influences the perception of the original experience and its recall. The actual memories and their meanings may thus bear little resemblance to the events and their meanings back in the past. Although an objective truth about the past may be impossible to discover, the actual process of remembering and discovering meaning is considered to be an intervention that leads to client improvement. For example, if a client reported a dream about incest and then doubted its veracity, the emphasis would not be on whether the incest occurred but rather on the truths inherent in the dream, on the conditions she experienced in her life that could have led to such a dream. Thus, the therapeutic intervention that involves the recovering of past memories generates its own truths if it is effective in terms of therapeutic benefit or progress.

In the constructivist tradition, radical behaviorists emphasize context and meaning. Take something out of context and it becomes meaningless. Put it in a new context, and it means something else; this is one of the reasons that Hayes (1987) prefers the term <u>contextualism</u> to radical behaviorism. <u>Problems—mental or otherwise—do not exist in isolation</u>. They are ascriptions of meaning that arise within a particular tradition, and have meaning only within that tradition. Even experiences that people consider purely physical are, in fact, shaped by language and previous experiences. Pain, for instance, is not simply the firing of nerve endings; it is part sensation, part fearful ideation—a package of interpretations surrounding sensations (Efran *et al.*, 1988).

Even though the contextualist (constructivist) position may be intellectually appealing, it is often difficult to bring these ideas into our lives in general, and into our psychotherapy practices in particular. That is, psychotherapists (radical behaviorists included) may accept contextualism on an intellectual level, but not on an emotional one. As expressed by Furman and Ahola (1988):

> We might, perhaps, when discussing philosophy with our colleagues readily agree that there is no one way of looking at things, but when it comes to our own beliefs about particular clients, we tend to cling tenaciously to our own truth. We forget that ideas are made up by observers and eventually convince ourselves that somehow they offer a blueprint of reality. . . . Why do we think we *know*, when in fact, we simply imagine, construe, think, or believe? (p. 30)

Nonmentalistic View of Behavior: The Focus on Environmental Variables That Control Behavior

Radical behaviorism explains human action in terms of behavior instead of entities or objects inside the brain. Thus, instead of "memory" and "thought," the analysis is based on "remembering" and "thinking." The behavior of putting a coin in a candy vending machine is seen as behavior and not as a mere sign that indicates the presence of some other nonbehavioral entity, such as drive, desire, expectancy, attitude, or a breakdown in ego functions. An adequate explanation would focus on those variables affecting the behavior, such as the number of hours without eating, and not on mental entities. In mentalism, inner psychological processes, such as "willpower," and "fear of failure," are given homuncular power to cause other, more behavioral events to come about. Explanations of behavior are incomplete if they do not involve tracing the observable antecedents of behavior back as far as possible into the environment. Many current psychological "explanations" do little more than specify some inner process as the cause of a particular aspect of behavior. It is only reasonable to ask what makes the inner process work as it does.

It is important to note that Skinner objects to things that are mental, not to things that are private. Private events, however, are not given any unique status other than their privacy. They are cut from the same cloth as is public behavior, and are subject to the same discriminative and reinforcing stimuli that affect all behavior. Thus, in Skinner's view, a client's private response can have as much or as little causal effect on subsequent behavior as a public one.

In seeking explanations of behavior then, radical behaviorists view themselves as essentially engaged in a search for "controlling variables." Events are considered controlling variables when they are perceived to be related to behavior in some way. Verbal behavior describing a relation between behavior and controlling variables is called the *statement of a*

functional relationship, and a systematic attempt to describe functional relationships is called a *functional analysis of behavior.*

Focal Interest in Verbal Behavior Controlled by Directly Observed Events

All verbal behavior, no matter how private its subject matter may
appear to be, has its origins in the environment. Although the phenomena related to human verbal functioning vary from the most intimately
personal to the most publicly social, all meaningful language is shaped
into effective form by the action of an environmental verbal community.
Thus, when a speaker says she sees an image in her mind's eye, what
is *said* must have been taught to her in childhood by others who could
not see into her mind's eye. These "teachers" must have used directly
observed events in the teaching process (see Chapters 4 and 6).

What sorts of factors are involved in leading the speaker to say what
he or she does? To know thoroughly what has caused a person to say
something is to understand the significance of what has been said in its
very deepest sense (Day, 1969). For example, to understand what a man
means when he says he just had an out-of-body experience, we would
search for its causes. First, we would want to know about the stimulation
in the body that was just experienced. Then, we would want to know
why a particular bodily state is experienced as out-of-body. Thus, we
would look for environmental causes going back into the man's history,
including the circumstances he encountered as he was growing up that
resulted in his saying "body," "out of," "just had," and "I." (A description of some of the experiences that result in "I" is given in Chapter 6.)
As soon as we knew all of these, then we would deeply understand the
significance of what was meant.

Direct observation is highly valued as a method of gathering relevant data. It is important to note, however, that what is observed does
not have to be public. Skinner is critical of the philosophy of "truth by
agreement," a perspective often adopted by conventional behaviorists
who claim that scientific knowledge must be essentially public in nature.
In fact, most of the time it is easiest to view observation as something
private because only one person can participate in a single act of observation. Similarly, interest is not restricted to events that are considered
to be observable in principle by someone else. Radical behaviorists feel
as free to observe or otherwise respond to their own reactions to a
Beethoven sonata as they are to observe those of someone else (Day,
1969). Once the observation of behavior has taken place, observers are
encouraged to talk interpretatively about what has been seen, recogniz-

ing that the particular interpretation that is made will be a function of their own special history. They merely hope that what they see will come to exert an increasing influence on what they say.

The increasing influence of the world on what is said is also referred to as increasing *contact* with the world. Contact is highly desirable in the scientist and can be viewed as the core of science. Improved contact is also desirable for most clients who are seen in psychotherapy. For example, the client who does not express emotions (see Chapter 4), also can be described as avoiding contact with situations that evoke emotions, and because of this would have difficulties in intimate relationships.

The above philosophical principles—that knowledge is contextual, behavior is viewed nonmentalistically, and that even the most private verbal behavior has its origins in the environment—have provided a language and concept of human nature intended to clarify the interaction between an individual's behavior and the natural environment. Radical behavioral concepts have been used to explain a wide range of therapeutic practices such as psychoanalysis and desensitization, as well as human experiences such as feeling, worrying, the self, and anger.

The application of Skinnerian concepts, termed *applied behavior analysis*, is a more narrow approach that uses analogies to operant conditioning procedures developed in the laboratory for solving real-life clinical problems. We use the term *analogies* because there are significant differences between clinical application and laboratory work (as discussed later), which have important implications for psychotherapy. In the following section, we will elaborate on how the conceptual foundations of applied behavior analysis form the theoretical underpinnings for FAP.

THEORETICAL UNDERPINNINGS OF FAP

The major focuses of applied behavior analysis are reinforcement, specification of clinically relevant behaviors, and generalization (Kazdin, 1975; Lutzker & Martin, 1981; Reese, 1966). These procedures have been extremely powerful in treating residents of hospitals, students in classrooms, and young or severely disturbed children—populations with whom the therapist exerts a great deal of control over the daily life environment. With the exceptions of Hayes (1987) and Kohlenberg and Tsai (1987), radical behaviorism and applied behavior analysis have been overlooked as a source for clinical procedures in the office treatment of adult problems.

The overlooking of radical behaviorism for ideas about doing adult psychotherapy is a bit of a mystery to us. As we have pointed out, the theory is comprehensive and encompasses many of the concepts that are important to the psychotherapist. The theory has also been around for some time. Many of the ideas relevant to psychotherapy were published in the 1950s (Skinner, 1953, 1957). There also are many individuals, the applied behavior analysts, who are both familiar with the theory and who are interested in clinical work. It is possible that the very success of applied behavior analysis within controlled environments (e.g., hospitals, schools) prevented its application to the less controlled psychotherapy environment. That is, the applied behavior analysts were so successful with a limited application of the theory that they did not pursue the broader implications of radical behaviorism relevant to adult psychotherapy.

An additional hindrance to the application of radical behaviorism comes from the difficulties in transferring the methods of applied behavior analysis to the psychotherapy setting. Constraints of adult outpatient treatment include therapist-client contact limited to one or more therapy hours per week, the therapist not observing the client outside the session, and lack of control over contingencies outside the session. FAP is based on the exploration of how reinforcement, specification of clinically relevant behaviors, and generalization can be accomplished within the constraints of the typical office treatment setting.

Reinforcement

Central to behavior analytic treatment is the direct shaping and strengthening of more adaptive repertoires of behavior through reinforcement. We use the term *reinforcement* in its technical, generic sense, referring to all consequences or contingencies that affect (increase or decrease) the strength of behavior. The definition of reinforcement is a functional one; that is, something can be defined as a reinforcer only after it has shown an effect in increasing or decreasing the strength of a behavior.

To some readers, however, this may not be a satisfying definition because it does not identify specific reinforcers such as ice cream, sex, or M&Ms. Reinforcement cannot be so defined because it is a process; an object becomes a reinforcer only in the context of the process and cannot be identified independent of it. Although ice cream may reinforce one person's behavior, it may have no effect on someone else's behavior, and therefore would not be a reinforcer for that behavior. Furthermore, reinforcement may not be something that we like. For example, a dentist being there for our dental appointment strengthens our behavior of making appointments even if the dental work itself is an unpleasant experience.

√In addition, it is important to note that reinforcement is an unconscious process; much of our behavior was shaped by the process of reinforcement before we even learned to talk. A physical change that we cannot feel occurs in our brain when reinforcement occurs. Although we may experience sensations of pleasure, or an inclination to act in a certain way, we do not feel the actual strengthening of our behavior. For example, if a boy says, "I love you" to his girlfriend, and she grins warmly and says, "I love you too," he may feel pleasure in his body and think "this is wonderful." But the pleasure is independent of the strengthening process itself at that moment. The thought, "this is wonderful," was the result of the pleasure in that he was describing the feelings to himself. His behavior was strengthened, and he also had these pleasurable feelings and thoughts. His awareness of the thoughts and feelings that accompany the reinforcement process is not at all necessary for his behavior to be strengthened.

Since the beginning of time, only those creatures whose behavior was strengthened by consequences could adapt to a changing environment and thereby survive. Thus, the reinforcement process is the result of evolution. As we shall elaborate later, it is a fundamental behavioral process that leads to consciousness, thinking, self, and the essence of human experience.

Time and Place of Reinforcement

A well-known aspect of reinforcement is that the closer in time and place the behavior is to its consequences, the greater will be the effect. Anyone who has delivered food pellets to a rat in a Skinner box has seen the deleterious effects that delaying the reinforcer can have on the behavior of the animal. The shaping process is effective, however, if the lever press and food pellet are in close proximity. Similarly, it is easy for the behavior therapist to reinforce and thus strengthen clients' relaxation skills while they occur in the office. That is, clients will readily relax in the office when requested to do so because the therapist is right there and directly reinforces the behavior. On the other hand, it is often a problem to get clients to relax as requested at home in between sessions because the therapist can only reinforce the behavior at the time the clients come in for their appointment.

The implication for outpatient office therapy is that the effects of treatment will be stronger if clients' problem behaviors and improvements occur during the session, where they are closest in time and place to the reinforcement. This is why FAP is a treatment for daily life problems that also occur during the therapy session. Examples of such problems include behaviors manifested as intimacy difficulties, including fears of abandonment, rejection, engulfment; difficulties in expressing feelings; inappropriate affect, hostility, sensitivity to criticism, social anxiety, and obsessive-compulsiveness. These terms are not intended to refer to mentalistic or inferred states but are used as general descriptive terms to give the reader an idea of the range of observable client behavior that could be evoked and changed under the appropriate conditions during therapy.

Another major feature of FAP, and one that is more problematic, is that improvements in the client's behavior that occur in the office should be immediately reinforced. The reinforcement of behavior during the session is problematic because the therapist's very attempt to make reinforcement immediate and contingent also may inadvertently make it ineffective and perhaps even counterproductive.

The problem in using reinforcement during treatment has come from imitating the methods of experimental behavior analysts. In order to achieve the goal of reinforcement that closely followed the response, applied behavior analysts, when doing clinical work, have used procedures that are analogous to those used in operant animal laboratory experiments. These clinicians took the rule "Give the food pellet immediately after the response" and literally transposed it to the clinical setting, as in "Deliver the M&M immediately after the child remains in his chair for 2 minutes." The purpose of the laboratory experiments, however, was to study the parameters of reinforcement, not to benefit the subject or to obtain generalization to his or her daily life.

The clinical implications of using the type of arbitrary reinforcement employed in laboratory settings as contrasted to the type that occurs in the natural environment has been discussed extensively by Ferster (1967, 1972b,c). Anticipating the dangers of using reinforcement in outpatient office therapy, Ferster warned that many of the common rewards used by applied behavior analysts—food, tokens, and praise—may be arbitrary. He saw this as a serious clinical problem since the arbitrarily reinforced behavior would only occur when the controller was present or if the client was interested in the particular reward being offered. As an example of arbitrary reinforcement gone awry, he cited the case of a mute autistic, who was treated by behavior analysts, and who ceased to speak when food was not present.

Natural versus Arbitrary Reinforcement

Given the drawbacks of arbitrary reinforcement, FAP is aimed at providing natural reinforcement for client improvements that occur during the session. Our suggestions for how to do this are in Chapter 2. The following comparisons will help highlight the distinction between the two types of reinforcement. Arbitrary and natural reinforcers differ on the four basic dimensions that follow.

1. *How narrow is the response class?* Arbitrary reinforcement specifies a narrow performance, whereas natural reinforcement is contingent on a larger response class. For example, an instructor who is using arbitrary reinforcement in teaching a dyslexic boy how to read is prone to being shortsighted and counterproductive. As is the case with anyone using arbitrary reinforcement for educational purposes, this teacher must decide which behaviors get reinforced and which get punished. He decides to punish the boy for reading a comic book instead of the text. The teacher is showing one of the drawbacks in using arbitrary reinforcement, that is, he is requiring a narrow response—reading the textbook—and has lost sight of the wider response class of reading in general. The natural reinforcement inherent to reading (such as that provided by the information or entertainment) reinforces a broad response class which includes reading comic books, racing forms, and the like. Thus, a danger in using arbitrary reinforcement is that it may inadvertently interfere with natural reinforcement and the attainment of the goal behavior.

2. *Is the required behavior in the individual's existing repertoire?* Natural reinforcement begins with a performance already in the individual's repertoire, whereas arbitrary reinforcement does not take into account one's existing repertoire to the same degree as does natural reinforcement. Such is the case when a mother criticizes her daughter's first sewing project for crooked seams and does not take into account her level of ability in sewing. That is, the mother is using the arbitrary reinforcement of criticism which entails her failing to recognize that her daughter was doing well for her skill level. In contrast, natural reinforcement would consist of the mother's appreciation of a usable article of clothing in this first sewing attempt, no matter what it looked like.

3. *Who does the reinforcement primarily benefit?* Arbitrary reinforcement produces behavior changes in the person being reinforced that uniquely benefit the person doing the reinforcing. No benefits have to be provided to the person subjected to arbitrary reinforcement. In fact, people often are harmed by arbitrary reinforcement. Adults who sexually abuse chil-

dren use arbitrary reinforcement (threats, praise, physical abuse) to obtain compliance. They often claim benefits to the child by saying, "the child wanted it," or "she was given lessons in sexuality and so it was for her own good." This argument is ludicrous; any adult who sexually uses a child does not do so because of the benefits to the child. In fact, sexual abuse can cause a wide variety of problems and specifically interferes with the natural reinforcement for sexual behavior found in consensual intimate relationships.

4. *How typical and reliable is the reinforcer in the natural environment for the behavior being exhibited?* Another way of posing this question is, "What is the reinforcement likely to be in the individual's natural milieu for this particular behavior?" Natural reinforcers are more fixed and stable parts of the natural milieux than are arbitrary ones. This is the most easily assessed aspect of reinforcement since an observer does not need to know the histories of the individuals involved in the reinforcement transaction to tell how typical the reinforcement is that is being used. For example, most people would agree that giving your son candy for putting on his coat is arbitrary, whereas his being chilled for being coatless is natural. Paying your daughter to practice the piano is arbitrary; whereas her playing simply because of the music created is natural. Similarly, fining your client a quarter for not making eye contact is arbitrary, while letting your attention wander is natural.

In sum, natural reinforcement is different from arbitrary reinforcement in that it strengthens a wide response class, takes into account the individual's skill level, benefits primarily the person receiving the reinforcement as opposed to the person giving it, and is typical and reliable in the natural environment. Most consequences, however, do not fit neatly into the categories associated with either arbitrary or natural reinforcement and probably have the dimensions of both.

Although no research has compared arbitrary and natural reinforcement directly, data that support our position paradoxically have been obtained from cognitively oriented research intended to discredit the behaviorist's emphasis on reinforcement. The research concerns the effects of external reward on intrinsic motivation (these are not behavioral terms but are those used by the nonbehavioral investigators). For example, Deci (1971), in a study typical of this type of research, paid one group of subjects for correct solutions to a puzzle and compared them to an unpaid group who were given the same puzzle. When left alone for eight minutes in a "free-time" situation, the paid subjects spent less time playing with the puzzle than the unpaid subjects. After reviewing the literature on such research, Levine and Fasnacht (1974) argued that "external rewards" are dangerous because they do not have much staying power (i.e., reduce resistance to extinction) and interfere with generalization, thereby "undermining" the very behavior they are aimed at strengthening. Operationally, "external rewards" and "intrinsic motivation" correspond to Ferster's notions of arbitrary and natural reinforcement. Although originally intended to demonstrate deficiencies in the behavioral approach, the intrinsic motivation data can be seen alternatively as an instance in which arbitrary reinforcement has negative effects.

Specification of Clinically Relevant Behavior

Second to reinforcement, behavior analysis is characterized by its attention to specification of the behaviors of interest. The term *clinically relevant behavior* (CRB) includes both problem behaviors and goal or target behaviors. We will discuss, in turn, the two components of the specification of clinically relevant behaviors—*observation* and *behavioral definition*—and the implications of specification for doing adult outpatient therapy.

Observation

Observation is a necessary precursor to behaviorally defining clinically relevant behaviors. Behaviorists assume that if the behaviors can be observed, they then can be specified and counted. Obviously, the client's problem behavior cannot be observed unless it occurs in the presence of the therapist. In order to meet this requirement, behavior analysts have either (a) treated clients who are restricted in movement, such as those who are in hospitals or prisons, or (b) treated problems that are severe, such as echolalia in autistic children, which occurs with high frequency.

Although it is convenient to use severe problems and restricted environments in order to directly observe the problem behavior, any problem that can be directly observed is adequate for a behavioral analysis. The outpatient psychotherapy environment fulfills this requirement if the client's daily life problem is of such a nature that it also occurs during the session. A salient, although trivial, example is someone who is seeking treatment for becoming tongue-tied when telling a doctor about problems, and who then actually becomes tongue-tied when telling the therapist about this problem. Thus, based on the observation requirement, a behavior analytic approach to outpatient therapy focuses on those problems in the outside world that also occur during the session.

Behaviorally Defining Clinically Relevant Behaviors

Traditionally, behavior analysts have used behavioral descriptions of target behaviors that refer only to observables. This requirement is for the purpose of obtaining reliability as measured by interobserver agreement. The observers, who must agree on whether a problem behavior has occurred, usually include the therapist and at least one other person. The other person(s) used as observers, however, as a matter of convenience, usually have been relatively inexperienced persons, such as undergraduates. Inexperienced observers can do the job when the behaviors of interest are straightforward, such as completing a math problem, a facial tic, or nail biting. Inexperienced observers are a problem when the behaviors are somewhat more complex (e.g., anxiety and marital discord). When the problem behaviors are more complex, training is required before the observers can do the job. The amount of training that can be done, however, is limited. Thus, the use of relatively naive observers has placed a practical limit on the complexity of the behaviors that the applied behavior analyst has worked with. For example, it would rule out treatments involving goal behaviors that are absent from the observers' repertoires and which cannot be remedied by observer training. Examples of such client behaviors include more subtle interpersonal reactions such as those related to intimacy and taking interpersonal risks.

In practice, it is almost impossible to achieve the desired objectivity based on the typical behavioral descriptions given for applied problems (Hawkins & Dobes, 1977). Interobserver agreement is greatly assisted, however, if the behavior being observed is in the repertoires of the observers. Although certain skills (e.g., basketball freethrows and gymnastics) can be reliably observed and evaluated by someone who cannot perform the skills, in general it is difficult to achieve reliability with more complex interpersonal behaviors if they are absent from the observer's repertoire. Consequently, it is easier for therapists to see and define clinically relevant behaviors if the goal behavior is in their own repertoire. For example, it might be difficult for a therapist who has not developed intimate relationships to discriminate the absence or presence of intimacy related behavior in the client.

Thus, direct observation and behavioral definition of problem and goal behaviors for the more subtle types of problems that adult psychotherapy clients present can be accomplished if (a) the problem-related behaviors occur during the session and thus can be directly observed and if (b) the therapist and observers are carefully selected so that they have in their own repertoires the client's goal behaviors.

Arranging for Generalization

Therapy is ineffective if the client improves in the therapy environment, but the gains do not transfer to daily life. Thus, generalization has been a primary concern for applied behavior analysts. The best way to arrange for generalization is to do the therapy in the same environment where the problem occurs. Historically, behavior analysts have accomplished this by delivering immediate reinforcement in institutions, classrooms, homes, or wherever else it was possible to provide treatment in the natural milieux where the problem occurred.

How does one measure or determine if two environments are similar? A formal analysis attempts to describe and compare the environments in terms of physical characteristics. The limitation of such an analysis is encountered when comparing two environments that are different in some ways but similar in others. For example, if you provide treatment for attention deficits in a special education classroom, will it generalize to a regular classroom or to the home environment? To avoid this problem, the comparison can be based on a functional analysis. Rather than looking at physical characteristics, the environments are compared on the basis of the behavior they evoke. If they evoke the same behavior, then they are functionally similar.

Although behavior analysis traditionally has not been done in the adult psychotherapy environment, it could be if the therapy environment were functionally similar to the client's daily life environment. A functional similarity between the natural and the therapy environment is indicated if clinically relevant behaviors occur in both settings. For example, a man whose presenting problem is hostility that develops in close relationships would show that the therapy environment is functionally similar to the daily life environment if he becomes hostile toward the therapist as their relationship develops.

In this chapter, we have laid the groundwork for functional analytic psychotherapy by describing its philosophical and theoretical assumptions. As we outlined in the preface, Chapters 2 and 3 are devoted to clinical technique and to ways of enhancing therapist awareness. Then, in Chapters 4 and 5, we reconceptualize the role and importance of memories, emotions, and cognitions in changing behavior. In Chapter 6, we formulate a behavioral theory of the development of the sense of self and discuss its clinical implications. In Chapter 7, we compare and contrast FAP with psychoanalysis and with behavior therapies, and explore how FAP capitalizes on the best features of the two approaches. Finally, ethical, supervisory, research, and cultural issues are examined in Chapter 8.

2

Clinical Application of Functional Analytic Psychotherapy

The clinical application of FAP will be discussed in terms of certain types of client behavior and therapist behavior, all of which occur during the therapy session. The client behaviors are his or her problems, improvements, and interpretations. The therapist behaviors are therapeutic methods that include evoking, noticing, reinforcing, and interpreting the client's behavior.

CLIENT PROBLEMS AND CLINICALLY RELEVANT BEHAVIORS

Everything a therapist can do to help clients occurs during the session. To the radical behaviorist, the therapist's actions affect the client via three stimulus functions: (1) discriminative, (2) eliciting, and (3) reinforcing. A *discriminative stimulus* refers to the external circumstances under which certain behaviors were reinforced and thus are more likely to occur. Most of our behavior is under discriminative control and is commonly known as *voluntary behavior* (operant behavior). An *elicited behavior* (respondent behavior) is produced reflexively and is commonly called *involuntary*. The *reinforcing function* (discussed in Chapter 1) refers to the consequences that affect behavior. Every action of the therapist has one or more of these three effects. For example, the therapist's action might be to ask, "What are you feeling right now?" The discriminative effect says, "It is now appropriate to say how you are feeling." The question, however, also might be aversive to the client and thus punish his or her behavior that immediately preceded the therapist's question; this is the reinforcing function. The eliciting function of the question might make the client turn red, sweat, and induce other private bodily states. The reasons the client reacts in these ways to the therapist's question about feelings are found in the client's history.

Since we assume that (1) the only way a therapist helps the client is through the reinforcing, discriminative, and eliciting functions of what the therapist does, and that (2) these stimulus functions within the session will have their strongest effects on client behavior occurring during the session, then the most important characteristic of a problem that makes it suitable for FAP is that it can happen during the therapy session. In addition, client improvements also must take place during the session and be naturally reinforceable by the reinforcers present within the session. Mainly, the reinforcers are the therapist's actions and reactions to the client.

Three client behaviors that can occur during the session are of particular relevance and are referred to as *clinically relevant behaviors* (CRB).

CRB1: Client Problems That Occur in Session

CRB1s are related to the client's presenting problems and should decrease in frequency during the course of therapy. Typically, CRB1s are under the control of aversive stimuli and consist of avoidance. Examples of such behavior that are actual instances of presenting clinical problems include the following:

1. A client whose problem is that she has no friends and "does not know how to make friends" exhibits these behaviors: avoids eye contact, answers questions by talking at length in an unfocused and tangential manner, has one "crisis" after another and demands to be taken care of, gets angry at the therapist for not having all the answers, and frequently complains that the world "shits" on her and that she gets an unfair deal.

2. A man whose main problem is that he avoids getting into love relationships always decides ahead of time what he is going to talk about during the therapy hour, watches the clock so he can end precisely on time, states that he can only come to therapy every other week because of tight finances (he makes $30,000 a year), and cancels the next session after making an important self-disclosure.

3. A self-described "hermit" who would like to develop a close re- lationship has been in therapy for three years and continues to muse periodically that his therapist is only in this for the money and is secretly contemptuous of him.
4. A woman who has a pattern of getting into relationships with unattainable men develops a crush on her therapist.
5. A woman who has a history of people leaving her because they "get tired" of her introduces new and involved topics at the end of the hour, frequently threatens to kill herself, and shows up drunk at her therapist's house in the middle of the night.
6. A man suffering from speech anxiety "freezes up" and is unable to talk to his therapist during the session.

CRB2: Client Improvements That Occur in Session

During the early stages of treatment these behaviors typically are not observed or are of low strength at those times when an actual in- stance of the clinical problem, CRB1, has occurred. For example, consider a client whose problem is withdrawal and accompanying feelings of low self-esteem when "people don't pay attention" to him during conversa- tions and in other social situations. This client may show similar with- drawal behaviors during a therapy hour in which the therapist does not attend to what he is saying and instead interrupts before he has com- pleted his sentence. Possible CRB2s for this situation include repertoires of assertive behavior that would have directed the therapist back to what the client was saying, or the discrimination of the therapist's waning interest in what was being said before the therapist actually interrupted.

The following case history illustrates the development of a client's CRB2s. Joanne was a bright, compassionate, and sensitive woman who came into therapy because she was troubled by constant anxiety, insom- nia, and recurring nightmares of rape. Although she suspected that when she was a child she had been sexually abused by her father, she had no specific memories of such abuse. She gradually improved in almost every aspect of her daily life over the 6 years that she worked with the second author. The following are some of the CRB2s that were strength- ened at various times during the treatment.

1. *Remembering and emotionally responding.* During Joanne's childhood, she experienced 10 years of unspeakable terror involving physical and emotional pain at the hands of someone who supposedly loved her, her father. Remembering and emotionally reacting to these events were not reinforced. Instead, forgetting and not emotionally reacting were func-

tional, and she avoided stimuli that could evoke undesired feelings. Her avoidance was pervasive, and in combination with the invalidating early experiences, she often felt devoid of a sense of self (see Chapter 6).

A major way that Joanne avoided reexperiencing such feelings as pain, terror, powerlessness, and rage was by avoiding intimate relationships. She was not open, trusting, or vulnerable. Thus, a therapeutic goal was to reduce generalized avoidance and increase the CRB2s of remembering and grieving. Gradually, Joanne was encouraged to increase her contact with vivid recollections of physical and sexual torture by her father—a process that was excruciatingly painful.

2. _Learning to ask for what she wants_ (i.e., that her needs were important and deserved attention). As with almost all survivors of sexual abuse, Joanne was reinforced for giving her father what he wanted but was severely punished for "wanting" for herself. She experienced this as not being entitled to expect from others and that "wanting" was "bad." I encouraged her to want and gradually, these CRB2s increased in strength. Thus, I attempted to reinforce any request that I could, such as those regarding topics discussed, the length and frequency of scheduled sessions, and verbal reassurances. In addition, Joanne was told that her needs were important and that if I or someone else did not meet them, it did not mean she was "bad" for having them. An important incident occurred about 4 months into her therapy, when she called me at 11:30 p.m. in the middle of a flashback. Joanne was panicked and shrieking. Since I recognized this call as a CRB2, I asked Joanne if she wanted to meet for a session right then; she said yes. Later Joanne told me it was very difficult for her to say yes, but she was terrified and really needed me to be with her. When I responded to her need, "wanting" was reinforced. Subsequently, Joanne learned to ask me for extra sessions and telephone time when she needed them, and this behavior of stating her wants and needs generalized to other relationships. As the strength of these CRB2s increased, there was a corresponding change in her feelings about "wanting" being acceptable and her needs being important.

3. _Trusting._ Because her father's reactions to her were erratic and unpredictable, Joanne was reinforced for anticipating and being hypervigilant for such behavior from significant others. She told me that it took six months of my always being on time for our appointments before she started believing that I would show up when I said I would. She stated, "I had all these fears—that you were going to think I was crazy, that you were going to hurt me, that my feelings were going to

scare you away. Rather than simply reassuring me, your response was to have me check out if that's what I was experiencing from you. I'd say no and you'd say you have to trust your experience." So Joanne gradually was less vigilant for an erratic action on my part which in turn allowed our relationship to grow. I was also reliable in keeping my word, consistent in the views I expressed, and did not behave unpredictably.

4. *Accepting love.* After some 3 years into therapy with me (she had been in therapy for 5 years prior to seeing me), Joanne described a daily life problem regarding her interpersonal relating. She said that deep inside she felt like she did not know how to love or be loved. I questioned her more, wanting to know exactly what she meant so that it could be viewed in behavioral terms. Joanne had difficulty describing it. In an attempt to see if it were happening in the session, I asked her if she could accept my love at the moment, and she said no, that she felt closed. Although it was a private process whose dimensions were difficult to describe, I judged that CRB1 was occurring at the moment.

T: How do you feel closed?

C: It feels like my heart is closed.

T: Totally closed?

C: It's about 5% open.

T: I'd like you to try to open it to 20% and take in my love for you.

C: It's about 25% open.

T: Great! Can you do 40%?

This process was maintained, and Joanne reported being able to "open her heart" more and more. Here is her description of what she experienced during that session: "It took courage to open up and draw in the love. It was a shift in focus in my mind and in my body. Although I was aware of my fear and the terror and pain of my experiences with my father, I focused on what I was feeling from you in the present as opposed to my fears. I let both be true—that my father had abused me, but that you were a person with whom I could feel safe and feel loved. I kept thinking to myself, 'I want to be open to taking in love.' I hold tension in my muscles when I shut down, a lot in my chest, like that muscle gets frozen. So the physical feeling of opening is softening that muscle, breathing more deeply, feeling the breath in my body. It's like the sensation of a lens aperture opening in my heart."

It is unclear what behavioral processes were involved with "accepting love," but Joanne's description of what she experienced suggests some possibilities. Our interpretation is that her not being able to accept love was a specific, largely private behavior which distanced her and reduced the aversiveness of relating to her father. Given some of the features of her description, some of these responses probably had been specifically evoked by the sexual abuse. Despite the aversiveness, she remained in contact with her feelings, and her avoidance extinguished, her physical responses changed, and there was an accompanying feeling of "accepting love."

That session was a significant turning point for Joanne because she learned she had control over whether she let love in or not. This aided in her developing more intimate love relationships.

CRB3: Client Interpretations of Behavior

CRB3 refers to clients' talking about their own behavior and what seems to cause it. It includes "reason giving" and "interpretations." The best CRB3s involve the observation and description of one's own behavior and its associated reinforcing, discriminative, and eliciting stimuli. The describing of functional connections can help in obtaining reinforcement in daily life. More details about this are given under Rule 5.

CRB3 repertoires also include descriptions of functional equivalence that indicate similarities between what happens in session and what happens in daily life. For example, Esther, a woman in her early forties, had not been sexually intimate with anyone for over 15 years. After 6 years in FAP with the second author, Esther became the lover of a man she met through church. Her CRB3 was, "The reason I'm in that intimate situation is because you had been there for me. It's such a phenomenal change. If not for you, I wouldn't be there. With you it was the first safe place I had to talk about what I feel, to find reasons why it's desirable to be sexual. There was a period of time that I was more overtly attracted to you, and you were accepting of my feelings. I learned that it was better to be whole and feel my sexuality than to be armored and empty, and I practiced learning how to be direct with you." This kind of statement can help increase transfer of client gains in the therapy situation to daily life. In this case, the behavior to be transferred helped increase the reinforcement obtained from being in a relationship.

Therapists sometimes confuse CRB3 repertoires with the behavior to which they refer. A client stating that she withdraws whenever she becomes dependent in a relationship (CRB3) is very different from actually withdrawing during the session because she is becoming dependent on the therapist (CRB1). It is also unfortunate that some therapists focus on those verbal repertoires that describe a problem behavior and fail to observe the problem behaviors (CRB1) or improvements (CRB2) as they occur.

Assessment

Initially, the assessment procedures of FAP are no different from those routinely used by therapists in clinical practice. The client is asked to report on problems and other conditions in his or her life. Interviews, self-reports, recorded material, questionnaires, and record keeping are used to define the problem, generate hypotheses about controlling variables, and monitor progress.

Once the therapist has some idea about the problem and its controlling variables, an assessment as to whether these are also occurring during the session is initiated. The therapist hypothesizes about whether a CRB1 is occurring at any particular moment, or presents a situation thought to be evocative of CRB1. These hypothesizing and evocative procedures are discussed in later sections.

FAP assessment then centers on one key question that the therapist continuously asks the client during treatment. "Is it happening now?" The "it" refers to CRB1. Variations are: "How are you feeling about yourself right now?" "Are you withdrawing right now?" "Is what just happened the same as the problem that brought you into treatment?" "Is the difficulty you have in expressing your feelings right now the same that you experience with your mother?" "What are you feeling right now . . . is it similar to the speech anxiety that brought you to therapy?"

FAP has no unique procedures for evaluating the validity of the client's self-report in response to the assessment question. On the one hand, the client's self-report is based on an event that just occurred— perhaps as little as two seconds before. It may, therefore, be less subject to distortions that time and distance can introduce into reported events that occurred in the past. On the other hand, the CRB1 is likely to have accompanying emotional responses that interfere with self-observation and also can be biased by the implied demand in the therapist's question. The advantage of assessing ongoing behavior, however, is that the therapist can directly observe the behavior that the client is describing. This allows for interobserver reliability assessments, the counting and recording of responses, and an opportunity to assess the correlation between verbal reports and the referent behavior.

THERAPEUTIC TECHNIQUE—THE FIVE RULES

Given that psychotherapy is a complex interactional process involving multidetermined behavior, our suggestions for therapeutic technique are not intended to be complete or to exclude the use of procedures not described here. Instead, other therapy methods can be complemented and augmented by assisting therapists in taking advantage of therapeutic opportunities that otherwise may go unnoticed. For example, the methods of cognitive therapy can be used along with FAP. FAP can augment cognitive therapy by providing additional therapeutic opportunities to work on irrational thoughts or faulty assumptions (see Chapter 5).

Our techniques are given in the form of rules. Rather than the rigid, threatening quality that is associated with common usage of this term, the rules we propose are based on Skinner's verbal behavior conception (1957, p. 339), with elaboration by Zettle and Hayes (1982). Within this context, the FAP rules are suggestions for therapist behavior that result in reinforcing effects for the therapist. It is more of a "try it, you'll like it" than "you'd better do it."

Furthermore, the rules do not give therapists specific guidance to cover every situation or moment during the therapy hour. It is expected that therapists will act in ways that depend on their experience and other theories. At the beginning of therapy, the time is usually spent on history gathering and obtaining descriptions of presenting problems. This may be followed by explorations with the clients as to how they could act to improve their situation. At any point during this process, the application of FAP rules can shift the focus of treatment to CRB. The focus may be momentary or may dominate the therapy. Thus, no procedures are ruled out, but at any moment FAP rule-governed technique could lead to the awareness and utilization of a therapeutic opportunity.

Rule 1: Watch for CRBs

This rule forms the core of FAP. Our major hypothesis is that following this rule improves therapeutic outcome, so the more proficient a therapist is at observing CRBs, the better will be the outcome. It is also hypothesized that following Rule 1 will lead to increased intensity; that is, stronger emotional reactions of the therapist and client to each other during the session.

In a therapy session, the primary consequence of client behavior is the therapist's reaction. Without clear observation of the client's behavior by the therapist, reactions can be inconsistent or antitherapeutic and progress will be compromised. In other words, if the therapist is not aware of the client's clinically relevant behaviors that occur during the session, reinforcement of improvements at the time they occur will be a hit-or-miss proposition. Although awareness or observation does not guarantee that improvements will be reinforced and that unfavorable behaviors will be extinguished or punished, it does increase the likelihood of appropriate therapist reactions.

The countertherapeutic problem caused by a lack of awareness is familiar to those who have worked with severely disturbed children. The first author recalls painstakingly teaching an in-patient child to put on his own socks—he had never done this before and it took about an hour a day for several weeks before this behavior was reliable. His parents came one morning to take him home for a visit and watched him get out of bed and put on his socks. I was beaming with pride at the child's accomplishment. But as soon as he had finished putting on both socks, his parents scolded him for putting on two different-colored socks and roughly pulled one off and replaced it with the right one. The client had a tantrum. Obviously, the parents did not observe the putting on of the socks as a CRB2, a member of the repertoire whose absence or low strength was directly related to the presenting problem. If the parents had been present during the tedious weeks of training, their awareness probably would have changed, and they instead would have naturally reinforced their son for having put on his socks. It is unfortunate that some psychotherapists often are unaware of their clients' clinically relevant behavior occurring during the session and are prone to react in an antitherapeutic manner, like the autistic child's parents.

As stated previously, the therapist is most likely to appropriately reinforce clinically relevant behavior occurring in the therapy situation if he or she observes it. Consider Betty, who was in treatment with the first author for speech anxiety, panic, and lack of assertiveness with male authorities, such as supervisors and executives, at her workplace. During the session, she asked me to call her physician and ask for a refill of her prescription for tranquilizers because she was too fearful of doing it herself. I had several strong, covert, negative reactions. First, since I am inclined to discourage medication use in favor of behavioral methods, I didn't like the idea. Second, I thought that getting a prescription refilled was Betty's responsibility, not mine. Third, I considered this as a chance for Betty to practice being assertive with her doctor. And fourth, calling her physician is an unpleasant task for me and I considered it an intrusion on my time. On the other hand, because of Rule 1, I was aware that this request itself was a CRB2, a clear cut within-session assertive response with a male authority, which heretofore was absent from Betty's repertoire. Given my awareness, I consented to call her doctor and complimented Betty on her forthrightness in making this request.

The importance of Rule 1 cannot be overemphasized. Theoretically, following Rule 1 by itself is all that is needed for successful treatment. That is, a therapist who is skilled at observing instances of clinically relevant behavior as they occur is also likely to naturally react to (reinforce, punish, extinguish) the client in a way that will foster the development of behavior useful in daily life.

Observing repertoires that include those specified by Rule 1 are highly developed in psychodynamic and eclectic therapists who are considered to be especially competent. This would be expected because those occurrences of CRB that are labeled *transference* serve as important discriminative stimuli in psychodynamically oriented treatment. In addition, most experienced therapists, regardless of theoretical orientation, would be expected to show Rule 1 types of behavior because awareness of CRB (even in the form of attending to transference issues) facilitates clinical improvements that automatically reinforce the psychotherapist's Rule 1 behavior. This reinforcement would be expected to take place without the therapist's awareness.

We believe the effects of Rule 1 are reflected in the results of a recent study on the outcome of psychoanalytic interpretations (Marziali, 1984). In this study, the interpretations made by the therapist were categorized into those that mentioned the client's behavior as it was occurring in the session (T interpretations), those that mentioned behavior occurring outside the session during daily life (DL interpretations), and those regarding behavior that occurred in the client's past (P interpretations). Client improvement was correlated with the number of T-type interpretations. From a FAP viewpoint, a T interpretation meant that the therapist was observing CRB (e.g., doing the same behavior called for by Rule 1). The more often CRB was observed, the greater was client improvement. In our view, improvements were derived from the contingencies provided by the therapist that tend to naturally occur once there has been observation. The interpretation itself could also have contributed to the improvement, but from a FAP standpoint, would be less important than the contingencies of the therapist's naturally reinforcing reactions to client improvements in the session.

Rule 2: Evoke CRBs

From our point of view, the ideal client-therapist relationship evokes CRB1 and provides for the development of CRB2. The degree to which this ideal is met depends, of course, on the nature of the client's daily life problems. It is possible that a distant, removed, blank screen of a therapist could be just right for some clients. A certain amount of passiveness could give the client a chance to develop independently (see Chapter 6 on the treatment of self problems). More generally, however, most clients need to learn how to have intimate relationships, which means that the therapeutic relationship should evoke client behavior that prevents intimacy from developing (CRB1). If the client's relationship skills are adequate for a passive and distant therapist, nothing about developing intimacy would be learned. A warm active therapist, on the other hand, could evoke the client's problems and set the stage for improvement. A client who wishes to have close relationships, and yet is frightened by warmth, can clearly benefit from a therapist who expresses warmth.

Client descriptions of what they want from the therapeutic relationship point to the importance of an evocative relationship. As one client stated, "Therapy is about building a loving relationship. If you can overcome your blocks with one person, you can go on to do it with others." Another client echoed similar sentiments, "If bad relationships messed me up, then it follows that I need good relationships to help me heal. And this is a good relationship."

Peck (1978) gave his view on what makes psychotherapy effective and successful:

> It is human involvement and struggle. It is the willingness of the therapist to extend himself or herself for the purpose of nurturing the patient's growth—willingness to go out on a limb, to truly involve oneself at an emotional level in the relationship, to actually struggle with the patient and with oneself. In short, the essential ingredient of successful deep and meaningful psychotherapy is love. (p. 173)

Greben (1981), whom we quoted at the beginning of the book, had a viewpoint similar to that of Peck:

> Psychotherapy is not a set of elaborate rules about what one may not do: rules about when to speak or not to speak, how to handle vacations, how to deal with missed hours, and so on. It is something much more simple than that. It is the meeting and working together of two people; it is hard honest work. You might say, it is a labor of love. (p. 455)

Our interpretation of the descriptions of Peck and of Greben is that the client learns from being involved in a real relationship. A therapist who loves, struggles, and is fully involved with a client provides a therapeutic environment that evokes corresponding CRB1.

In addition to the general approach taken by the therapist, there are other ways the environment can be structured to evoke CRB. Although not intended, specific therapeutic techniques used by various psychotherapists might be effective because they evoke CRB. Some examples are (1) _free association_, which can be viewed as presenting an unstructured task that calls for introspection and would evoke related CRB (see Chapter 6); (2) _hypnosis_, which can evoke CRB related to giving up control; (3) _homework assignments_, which can evoke countercompliance or excessive compliance-related CRB; (4) _imagery exercises_, which can evoke CRB related to being constricted, creative, or emotional. Cognitive restructuring, talking to empty chairs, reporting dreams, and primal screaming no doubt evoke CRB1s appropriate for some clients. The problem with these techniques is that the therapist who uses them may be so intent on looking for alter egos, wise men within, unconscious material, and dysfunctional cognition, that the CRB evoked is not seen or is viewed as incidental.

Other approaches include (1) requesting that a spouse attend the sessions if repertoires relevant to the client's relationship problems only emerge when the spouse is present (couples counseling), (2) beginning a session with a bulimic eating lunch if the CRBs occur only after a meal has been eaten, and (3) withholding comments that convey acceptance or approval of the client for a period of time if the CRB concerns the client's difficulties relating to people who are not explicit about their approval and acceptance.

The last example given raises a problem that can occur when a therapist deliberately alters an aspect of his or her behavior in order to increase the chances of obtaining CRB. The therapist can go too far in setting up conditions to evoke CRB and his or her credibility can become jeopardized because of the nature of such arbitrary reinforcement. For example, a therapist may feign anger in order to evoke CRB in a client whose difficulties are provoked by people who get angry. Even though the feigned anger can result in an important therapeutic interaction, the client may come to recognize that the anger was not really anger but instead was performed for the benefit of the client. Subsequent therapist anger then could be viewed, justifiably, as a ruse and thereby not serve to evoke CRB. Further, the client may come to distrust therapist affective expressions or statements. Needless to say, such an outcome would seriously hamper progress.

The situation described above needs to be differentiated from one in which a client's presenting problem is a lack of trust that interferes with important relationships. Such distrustfulness did not originate from interactions with the therapist as in the example cited, but instead has a long history, and its occurrence in the therapeutic relationship is consistent with this history. In such a case, doubting the sincerity of the therapist's reactions constitutes a CRB and should be a focus of treatment. It would be particularly unfortunate if a therapist strengthened mistrust in such a client through a misguided attempt to set up conditions in order to provoke CRB. A safeguard that might help prevent mistrust would be to explain to the client why the therapist is altering his or her behavior before actually doing so.

Rule 3: Reinforce CRB2s

It is difficult to put Rule 3 into practice. The only natural reinforcers available in the adult therapy situation are the interpersonal actions and reactions between client and therapist. On the one hand, reinforcement that is close in time and place to the goal behavior is the primary change agent available in the therapeutic situation. On the other hand, behaviorists who are aware of the importance of reinforcement are prone to use procedures that are arbitrary and thereby risk compromising their effectiveness. As Ferster (1972a) stated, "natural reinforcers are sometimes puzzling because they seem to reinforce so much behavior and yet their effects appear to be evanescent when there is an attempt to use them deliberately" (p. 105).

There are direct and indirect approaches to providing natural reinforcement. The direct approaches consist of what a therapist can do at the moment that a reinforcer is called for; however, they carry a larger risk of producing arbitrary reinforcement. The indirect approaches enhance the occurrence of natural reinforcement by manipulating variables other than what one does immediately after the behavior and carry a smaller risk of being arbitrary.

Direct Approaches

Quite clearly a therapist who plans to say "good client" or displays exaggerated reactions whenever a reinforcer is called for runs the risk of being arbitrary. This is probably why Wachtel (1977) said that behavior therapists were overly exuberant in their use of praise, which "cheapened" the interaction. Deliberate attempts to reward an adult client, which is guided by such a rule as "when the client shows an improvement make a positive gesture or pay a compliment," could easily lead to arbitrary reinforcement. So, as a general guideline, it is advisable to avoid procedures that attempt to specify the form of the therapist reaction in advance. Specifying the form of the therapist response seems to happen whenever one attempts to conjure up a reinforcing reaction without relating it to the specific client-therapist history. For example, if you were to try to think of what you could say to a client that would be reinforcing, such phrases as "that's terrific" or "good" come to mind. These specific forms of response could easily be arbitrary because they were thought of outside the context of the client-therapist environment at the moment of reinforcer delivery.

1. *Reinforce a wide response class in clients.* Having a wide response class in their repertoires is more naturally reinforcing for clients because it tends to be generalizable to many other situations. Take the case of a male obsessive-compulsive client whom the therapist is encouraging to loosen up in his dealings with family and friends. He gradually starts coming late to sessions, tries to stay overtime, and lets his bill become past due. A narrow response called for would dictate that he be called to task, whereas seeing his new, less responsible behaviors as progress (CRB2s) would reinforce a wider response class in him.

2. *Match your expectations with the clients' current repertoires.* This means being aware of your client's current skill level in whatever changes he or she is trying to make (e.g., communicating better, describing feelings, controlling impulses), and not making your expectations too high. The concept of shaping can help in being aware of current repertoires. For example, the second author was seeing a client named Agnes, diagnosed as "borderline" according to DSM-III-R, who was moody, explosive, and verbally abusive. Often, she would abruptly terminate therapy without prior notice and without any apparent provocation. These were the same problems Agnes was having in her daily life, and had led to only short stints of previous therapy with numerous therapists because they would find her intolerable.

After a year of therapy, during which I had showed an unusual amount of patience and tolerance for this behavior, Agnes once again terminated, threatened suicide, and stated she was doing this because I cared little about her needs as indicated by the limited time I was willing to spend with her. Although I could have viewed this as the last straw, the concept of shaping helped in the discrimination of this event as a potential CRB2 which should be reinforced. Agnes was, for the first time, describing external variables as the cause of her outburst before storming out of the office. I reinforced this improvement by talking to her about how I could better meet her needs, and negotiated with her the length and frequency of our sessions. Through shaping, Agnes's anger and abusiveness decreased over time, and were replaced by direct requests and descriptions.

3. *Amplify your feelings to increase their salience.* Sometimes it is helpful to add other verbal behavior to a basic reaction to the client in order to ensure or increase therapeutic effectiveness. Although the nature of the reinforcer is not fundamentally changed in this process, amplification can be therapeutically important. This process is manifested in a therapist's being especially careful in explaining reactions to the client as well as in describing private or weak reactions that may not be immediately discernible.

To illustrate, consider a case in which a client who has intimacy concerns and lacks friends behaves in a way that results in some private, spontaneous reactions in the therapist. These responses may include (1) predispositions to act in intimate and caring ways, and, (2) private respondents that correspond to "feeling close." Because these probably are not discriminated by the client or have weak reinforcing effects, the therapist could describe the private reaction and say, "I feel especially close to you right now." Without amplification, such important basic reactions would have little or no reinforcing effects on the client's behavior that caused it.

4. *Be aware that the relationship exists for the benefit of the client.* Whatever interventions are made, it is important to constantly keep in mind the question, "What is best for my client at the moment and in the long run?" As a means of further illustrating this principle, we will explore the relationship between the concept of natural reinforcement and the type of therapy advocated by Carl Rogers. Although Rogers espoused a much different approach than that in FAP, the characteristics of a naturally reinforcing therapist are in some ways reminiscent of Rogers's caring and genuineness. Known for his opposition to "using reinforcement" to control other people, Rogers would certainly not "try" to use it. Yet a careful analysis of his reactions to clients indicates that contingencies exist (Truax, 1966) because Rogers reacted differentially to certain classes of client behavior. Thus, caring and genuineness produce a pattern of reinforcement.

From our point of view, Rogers's caring probably manifested itself as particular interest, concern, distress, and involvement that ended up naturally punishing CRB1s and reinforcing CRB2s and CRB3s. Thus, we suggest that Rogers's call for genuineness and caring is an indirect method of enhancing the occurrence of naturally reinforcing contingencies. A therapist who cares, according to the present formulation, is one who naturally reinforces or is governed by what is best for the client.

Since the therapy relationship is one of unequal power, it is especially important to keep this guideline in mind. Otherwise, clients can

ploited and harmed. Clients who engage in sex with their
e a case in point. Peck (1978) wrote an excellent discussion
difficult to conceive of the client's benefiting from sexual
th a therapist:

> Were I ever to have a case in which I concluded after careful and judicious
> consideration that my patient's spiritual growth would be substantially fur-
> thered by our having sexual relations, I would proceed to have them. In fifteen
> years of practice, however, I have not yet had such a case, and I find it difficult
> to imagine that such a case could really exist. First of all, the role of the good
> therapist is primarily that of the good parent, and good parents do not con-
> summate sexual relationships with their children for several very compelling
> reasons. The job of a parent is to be of use to a child and not to use the
> child for personal satisfaction. The job of a therapist is to be of use to a patient
> and not to use the patient to serve the therapist's own needs. The job of a
> parent is to encourage a child along the path toward independence, and the
> job of a therapist with a patient is the same. It is difficult to see how a therapist
> who related sexually with a patient would not be using the patient to satisfy
> his or her own needs or how the therapist would be encouraging the patient's
> independence thereby. (p. 176)

5. *Atypical reinforcers, if used at all, should be transitional.* Occasionally,
a therapist may want to use atypical reinforcers in a transitional phase
of treatment until natural reinforcers take over. This should be done,
however, with great caution. Moreover, it would be helpful to explain
to the client why this is being done and that it should be phased out
and replaced with natural reinforcement. Ferster (1972b) proposed that
some of the successes of atypical reinforcers such as food or praise re-
inforcements are due to "the way they make the [client's] behavior more
visible to the [therapist] and the [client] himself." Once this awareness
has occurred, naturally reinforcing reactions on the part of the therapist
would prompt relevant repertoires in the client that accompany the arbitrary reinforcers.

For example, consider a client with a high absenteeism rate at work
and in therapy. Obviously, without contact it is difficult to develop a
therapeutic alliance. Surprises in the form of inexpensive tangible rewards, such as erasers, pencils, notebooks, and little toys, can be offered
as an inducement to regularly attend appointments. As v repertoires
develop that make the therapy itself sufficiently reinforcing, these rewards can be phased out.

6. *Avoid using punishment.* Consistent with the radical behavioral bias
against aversive controls, the emphasis so far has been on positive reinforcement. Aversive stimuli should be used only when positive reinforcement approaches are ineffective. The bias against therapeutic use

of aversive stimuli is based on its problematic side effects: (1) it can lead to avoidance of the therapy, (2) it can lead to general aggressiveness, and (3) it substitutes avoidance and escape for productive behavior. Ferster pointed out that most aversive control that occurs between people is arbitrary in nature. Thus, it makes sense to avoid, whenever possible, the use of aversive control in the office treatment of adults.

There are instances, however, when the client CRB1s consist of avoidance or escape behavior that precludes the occurrence of CRB2s—the development of more effective repertoires. In such instances, the therapist might attempt to block the avoidance by re-presenting the aversive SD that originally evoked the escape or avoidance. Consider, for example, this simple question asked by the therapist, "How did your relaxation practice go during the week?" after the client had agreed to practice daily. For some clients the question could be an aversive stimulus, and it would evoke avoidance or escape by changing the topic, lying, or giving an ambiguous response.

These reactions (e.g., not giving a straight answer) could be related to a wide range of presenting problems related to ineffectiveness in interpersonal relationships. If the therapist dropped the topic and went on to something else, the avoidance CRB1 would be reinforced and a significant client repertoire with far-reaching ramifications, "being direct," would not develop. Thus, the main technique for weakening avoidance CRB1s is to re-present the aversive stimulus which, for the above example, means repeating the question, "How did your relaxation practice go during the week?"

It is our impression that CRB1 avoidance behavior frequently occurs, possibly during every session. The therapist can always ask oneself, "What does the response avoid?" It is difficult to detect avoidance because the aversive situation can be highly idiosyncratic and thereby obscure to the therapist. In the above example, for instance, the client might start the session by bringing up a crisis even before the therapist asks the question about relaxation. The crisis may or may not be avoidance of the relaxation homework issue. Unless the therapist had formulated hypotheses about CRB1s related to the assignment of homework, the crisis would be a successful avoidance. The notion of avoidance, incidentally, from a functional standpoint often has little to do with the client's awareness and is primarily a contingency-shaped behavior. As pointed out earlier, the effects of any contingency can strengthen (or weaken) a behavior and has nothing to do with the client's awareness of the contingency (see Chapter 5 for further discussion of awareness and contingency-shaped behavior).

It is not advisable to block each and every escape or avoidance response because blocking is aversive control and carries all of the associated untoward effects. Correspondingly, it should be applied sparingly in the context of a primarily positive reinforcing environment and in accordance with the client's current level of toleration for aversive stimulation. Toleration refers to a decreased reaction and disruptive effect of the aversive stimulation. Toleration is increased through the positive reinforcement resulting from new behavior that develops after the initial aversiveness associated with a blocked avoidance. A verbal repertoire corresponding to the controlling variables involved in the avoidance (Rule 5) may also help to increase tolerance. An example of this would be, "I'm going to ask you again about the relaxation because you didn't answer. I'm doing this because I think your not answering is like what you do when your wife asks about your day and you both end up feeling angry. This may be an opportunity to do something about that problem."

7. *Be yourself as much as possible within the constraints of the therapy relationship.* One characteristic of natural reinforcement is that it occurs in the community. The therapist, as a member of the verbal community, has access to the natural reinforcers contingent on a particular client behavior that occurs during the session. To access these natural reinforcers, the therapist can observe the spontaneous private reactions that occur immediately after the client behavior. Technically, the private reaction *per se* is not naturally reinforcing; rather, it is accompanied by dispositions to overtly act in ways that are naturally reinforcing. Another method is to ask oneself, "How would the community respond to this behavior?" Neither can ensure that the reinforcer accessed is natural or that it is therapeutic, but it is a starting point. Three factors should be taken into account in determining whether the therapist's private reactions are likely to be naturally reinforcing: (1) awareness of the client's current repertoire, (2) awareness of the client's best interests, and (3) the therapist's having the goal repertoires.

Indirect Approaches

Thus far, we have discussed direct approaches to increasing the natural reinforcement of client behavior during the therapy session. As pointed out earlier, using a direct approach is risky. That is, when the therapist is following a rule about what to do at the time of reinforcement, it may become arbitrary because the rule is not part of the process when it occurs in the natural environment. For example, a good parent will usually act for the child's benefit without having to follow a rule about (be aware of) what they should do. Indirect approaches, on the other hand, are intended to aid in natural reinforcement by manipulating variables other than what one does immediately after noticing the CRB. For example, most therapists make sure they are not famished or exhausted during the session by eating and resting appropriately beforehand. This can be viewed as an indirect means of increasing the likelihood that the therapist will naturally reinforce client improvements. Consequently, eating and resting will help to ensure that the therapist will be more attentive, patient, and understanding and thus be more naturally reinforcing.

1. *Increase awareness of what to reinforce.* It is important to remember that improvements may come in many different forms and paces; increasing awareness of what to reinforce is the behavior called for in Rule 1, and is the most important of the indirect methods. The chances that a therapist's spontaneous reactions will be naturally reinforcing are improved if the client's behavior is discriminated as a clinical improvement.

2. *Assess your impact.* The general idea is to review therapeutic interactions in detail. Video and audio tapes would be helpful for this process as would having others observe the session (as occurs in teaching clinics). This feedback can help to change the therapist's reactions in a favorable way (Rule 4).

3. *Do good deeds that benefit others in general.* Another approach is for the therapist to engage in behavior in which the only conceivable reinforcer (for the therapist's behavior) is the benefit it provides to someone else. Suggestions include: increase the number of good deeds for strangers; do volunteer work; give to the poor and the hungry and other needy individuals. Do it frequently, perhaps every day. The hope is that this will strengthen repertoires for benefiting others which, in turn, is one of the defining characteristics of natural reinforcement. If this strengthened repertoire transfers into the therapy session, then it will help to increase the natural reinforcement available and thus lead to better therapy.

4. *Select clients appropriate for FAP.* Since FAP requires that the natural reinforcement available in the therapy situation be relevant to the clients' problem-related behaviors, a fourth approach that indirectly enhances the occurrence of natural reinforcement is the selection of clients who are likely (a) to have problems which occur during the session, and (b) to be affected by the therapist's reactions.

Rule 4: Observe the Potentially Reinforcing Effects of Therapist Behavior in Relation to Client CRBs

Rule 4 is directly derived from behavior analytic principles that stress the importance of the effects of the consequences of behavior on the future probabilities of that behavior. Although a change in the therapist's behavior can be a natural by-product of following this rule, the rule itself only specifies the therapist's observation of the reinforcing relationship between client-therapist behavior and does not suggest that the therapist intentionally alter his or her own behavior. The observation of the reinforcing relation can have important effects on therapeutic outcome. For example, the therapist's observation that his or her reactions appear to be punishing the client's low-strength desirable behavior can lead to changes in the therapist's behavior that will be positively reinforcing. It is also possible, however, that the therapist can continue to punish favorable behavior even after observing the antitherapeutic nature of the punishment. The outcome in this case could be a decision to refer the client to another therapist, or for the therapist to enter personal therapy aimed at altering those particular behaviors.

The therapist's observation of the reinforcing effects of his or her reactions on the client's behavior can help in following Rule 5 and in developing similar behaviors in the client—CRB3. The most obvious way this occurs is when the therapist tells the client about the self-observation: "I've noticed that each time you started talking about your spiritual beliefs I've changed the topic and you no longer bring it up." Thus, the therapist models making a statement of a functional relationship for the client.

Rule 4 can also lead the therapist to search for ways of enhancing the effects of reactions that could be reinforcing of CRB but that are not noticed by the client. For example, consider a male client who has had trouble expressing feelings because of a history of being ridiculed or criticized when he did so. He did not increase these behaviors even though the therapist listened intently with empathic facial reactions and softly spoken comments each time the client expressed a feeling. Inquiries led to the discovery that the therapist's reactions were not discerned by the client because the act of expressing feelings evoked such intense emotions (collateral private respondents) that outside stimulation was not noticed. After the therapist amplified the empathic reaction by speaking loudly and clearly, the client's rate of feeling expression appeared to increase.

It is advisable to avoid starting treatment if it seems likely that natural contingencies do not favor improvement for a particular client. Such is the case when Rule 4 leads the therapist to conclude that most of the reactions to a client will be punitive and these negative reactions are not related to the client's presenting problem, such as "people react negatively to me." The therapist may recognize that he or she does not like the client for reasons that are unlikely to change soon (e.g., the client reminds the therapist of a cruel foster parent or of a spouse who ran off with a lover last week).

Rule 5: Give Interpretations of Variables That Affect Client Behavior

Our hypothesis is that the behavioral interpretations called for by Rule 5 will help to generate more effective rules (Zettle & Hayes, 1982) and increase contact with controlling variables. These points are discussed later in more detail.

When asked, "Why did you do that," we respond with a reason or interpretation. Usually the reason includes a description of what we did (or thought, or felt, or saw) and a statement about the causes. What we did and what we say about the causes depends, of course, on our personal histories. Similarly, a psychotherapist's observations and interpretations of behavior are a function of history, including his or her clinical and theoretical background. Regardless of who gives it, however, a reason is just a bit of verbal behavior—a series of words. Nevertheless, every form of psychotherapy seems to include teaching the client to give reasons that are acceptable to the therapist. Specifically, the cognitive therapist teaches clients to give reasons for their problems and improvements in terms of their beliefs or assumptions, whereas the FAP therapist expects reasons in terms of a reinforcement history and current controlling variables. The psychoanalytic client, on the other hand, might give reasons in terms of childhood conflicts and repressed memories. The pervasiveness of reason-giving in psychotherapy is illustrated by the Woolfolk and Messer (1988) description of psychoanalysis as a process in which the client tells what happened and gives reasons which the analyst then restates (interprets), giving a different reason. Analysis is complete when the client's reasons are the same as the analyst's.

As therapists, we hope that the reasons that we give to our clients will help in daily life problems. Depending on the reason given and the client's history, however, it may actually have no effect or even hinder the client. Our view is that there are two ways that reason-giving can affect the client.

First, the reason can lead to a prescription, instruction, or rule. The interpretation, "You are acting toward your wife like you did toward your mother" can easily be taken as a prescription or rule that the client hears as, "Don't be so unfair to your wife; treat her differently since she obviously is not your mother. And if you treat her fairly, your marital relationship will improve." Whether or not the rule or instruction helps depends on how well it corresponds to the natural environment. For example, consider two reasons that might be given by a little girl who took a cookie when she was not supposed to. One reason might be, "The devil made me take the cookie." This reason does not correspond to environmental conditions that affected her cookie taking. On the other hand, the reason, "I took it because I haven't had a cookie in over a week" corresponds to environmental events. The latter reason suggests possible interventions (e.g., allowing her to have cookies more often) which could affect cookie stealing.

Second, a reason can enhance the salience of (increase contact with) controlling variables and increase positive and negative reinforcement density (Ferster, 1979). An analogy from animal research can illustrate this principle. Rats were placed for a period of time in two distinctive shock chambers from which there was no escape. In one chamber, non-contingent shocks were delivered at random intervals. In the other chamber, the same number of noncontingent shocks were given but each shock was preceded by a warning light. When given a choice, rats invariably preferred the signaled shock chamber. The same holds true for signaled and unsignaled food. The rats' choices indicated that a signal helped to improve their experience. Similarly, an interpretation could "signal" events for humans.

For example, a female client learns during FAP that the reason she feels rejected at times during the session is a function of the therapist's attentiveness and, further, this attentiveness is related to how harried or rushed the therapist appears at the beginning of the session. This interpretation could increase the client's noticing the therapist's mood at the beginning of the session and significantly affect the client's experience of a lapse in the therapist's attention. As a result, the client is in better contact (she notices how harried the therapist is), and then experiences less aversiveness when he is inattentive.

Statements of Functional Relationships

The verbal repertoire to be developed by therapists involves statements that relate events during the session to the relationship symbolized by $Sd\ R \rightarrow Sr$. This represents operant behavior in which (1) Sd is the discriminative stimulus or prior situation whose influence over the occurrence of R varies with the reinforcement history; (2) R is the response or operant behavior which is influenced by the *Sd*, and (3) *Sr* is the reinforcement or effect of the response on the environment.

For example, "When I asked you how you felt about me (the *Sd*), you responded by talking about your jail experience (the *R*), which is another topic that you know I'm interested in. I rewarded your avoidance by getting into discussing jail and not your feelings about me (the *Sr*)." Usually, it is preferable to make the statement in everyday language but it could be argued that it is valuable to teach behavioral language to the client. Statements regarding parts of the functional relationships, however, are better than none at all (e.g., "Whenever I ask about your feelings toward me [*Sd*], you change the topic [*R*]").

Rule 5 repertoires that correspond to behavior occurring in the session are preferred to those corresponding to events occurring elsewhere. But better still are verbal repertoires that relate controlling variables occurring outside the session to those occurring in the session because generalization is enhanced.

In the following case we illustrate the use of Rule 5. Andi, a lesbian of color in her twenties, came into therapy with the second author because she wanted to "change old patterns that prevent me from getting close to people." Initially, she had difficulty in talking about her feelings and in showing any kind of affect during therapy and reported similar behavior elsewhere. About 6 months into her therapy, in between sessions Andi spontaneously started writing me notes with more affective expression. Given Andi's paucity of expression during the sessions, I was delighted, read the notes, and responded to them. The notes increased in frequency and length. I was aware (Rule 1) of the possibility that the notes were a step in the right direction in terms of developing intimate relating (CRB2) and that the content of the notes included descriptions of controlling variables (CRB3).

After about a year of therapy she wrote, "I'm starting to feel scared about how dependent I'm getting. I can't imagine not having you in my life. It's one thing to become dependent on therapy, it's worse to become dependent on a particular person, a particular therapist. After all, there are lots of therapists out there, but not that many Third World feminists with left-of-liberal politics and an understanding of the lesbian community who like the way I write."

The following conversation occurred in the subsequent session:

T: Those are all true, but you left out that our relationship is special and unique and that I really care about you. (I was aware that this is a discriminative stimulus [*Sd*] for the type of intimate relating behavior that Andi lacked

[CRB2] as well as one that evokes avoidance and consequent difficulties in maintaining close relationships [CRB1]).

C: Lots of people care about me, but those characteristics set you apart. (Andi responded in such a way that I felt discounted; I was probably in the position that other would-be intimates had found themselves when they expressed caring—a CRB1).

T: I feel discounted when you say that.

Andi was visibly upset by this reaction. I then described important aspects of the functional relationship, "Andi, when I told you that I really care about you and wanted you to acknowledge my feelings, you reacted in an impersonal way. This reaction punished my telling you that I care and made me feel like my feelings don't count. I think that's why you reacted the way you did, that is, you don't want me to bring up my caring and positive feelings about you."

Andi elaborated on this theme and described how, in general, it was hard for her to hear messages from others which are caring, complimentary, or sensitive to her feelings—a pattern which interferes with her getting close to people.

Emphasis on Behavioral Processes

As a general strategy, the therapist reinterprets client statements in terms of functional relationships, a learning history, and behavior. Such behavioral interpretations emphasize history and downplay mentalism and nonbehavioral entities. This is useful to the client because it directs attention to external factors that lend themselves to therapeutic interventions.

For example, Angela, who was in treatment with the first author, lacked self-confidence, had poor self-esteem, felt unsure of herself in relationships, and had difficulty in asking others what she wanted from them.

C: I feel like I don't have a right to exist. Like I shouldn't really exist, like I'm just so much trouble. I think to myself, you know, I was such a mouse, I really was. Like when I learned to drive, four-way stops just petrified me cause I was scared to take my turn. I was afraid I was never supposed to go. It's still a little traumatic, but I've got it down now, but that must indicate something is wrong. Well, now what? [long pause] (Most of these descriptions, and particularly the four-way stop, could indicate how Angela felt now, in the relationship with me. See Chapter 3 on analyzing client verbal behavior.)

T: I don't know. I can tell you my thoughts or you could pick a direction to go in. (I am offering to amplify my private reactions.)

C: Well, I don't have a direction.

T: Do you want me to tell you what my thoughts are?

C: Or you could pick a direction. (Facial expression and voice tone indicate she does not want to hear my thoughts.)

T: That's true, I could pick a direction. But it seems that the idea of me telling you what my thoughts are is not attractive to you. That you don't like that idea. Can you say more about this? (Angela's avoidance of me telling my thoughts is a CRB1 because it is related to the difficulties she has in maintaining close relationships.)

C: Well, I guess it's just sort of . . . I guess it just doesn't . . . it's just not my policy. You know? Well, I just sort of cruise around, and I guess I don't get too . . .

T: personal?

C: (nods yes) Mm-hm. I guess I sort of rather stay on the surface.

T: Now did anything come to mind for you when I said I could tell you my thoughts? Did any ideas flash through your mind?

C: Well, sort of a dumb one. I guess it's sort of like it's one of these little danger points, you know. I just kind of back off. I guess I don't think it's a good idea. Well, I mean, sometimes it's a good idea, I guess, but not usually. Well, maybe sometimes. I guess I don't want to ask that question. (A description of an aversive Sd and the CRB1 of avoidance of getting too close, trusting, listening to what others may want.)

T: Mm-hm. OK, well, let me tell you what my thoughts are. When you said that you don't have the right to exist, it reminded me of how your mother was so upset about you falling in the creek because it was trouble for her. It was just one more example of her teaching you that you don't have the right to exist—to cause anybody any trouble. (An interpretation based on learning history and restating "no right to exist" in terms of not engaging in behaviors that cause people trouble.)

T: We run up against that in here when you really don't want me in any way to be troubled or go out of my way for you or to try and accommodate you in any way. That also is like coming up to the four-way stop. You don't want others to have to wait. If they want to go, they should be able to go. (Drawing a parallel between daily life and the client-therapist relationship and indicating the contingency of avoiding making trouble.)

T: So that's kind of one idea that I thought about as something that you run into. And then the other thing that I was thinking about is my high regard that I have for you. I mean, it's super high. I really, really think you're wonderful, and yet even though I've let you know this, it doesn't seem to impact you. I think your not wanting to know my thoughts has something to do with that. You are somehow not in full contact with that. That's your policy. So those are my thoughts. (This starts out with amplification of private behavior and brings into the therapy session a daily life situation of receiving positive feedback and caring from others but not being very influenced by it. It also is an attempt to restate the problem in behavioral terms—a hard-to-describe avoidance behavior. The interpretation can be taken as a covert rule: "It doesn't make sense to respond to me like you did to your mother.")

C: Well, okay, so given I should believe you, and not my mother, I don't know how to do that. (It would be appropriate here to give a behavioral interpretation of her experience of "not knowing how to do it" corresponding to the difference between contingency-shaped and rule-governed behavior as discussed in Chapter 5. The interpretation would emphasize that the problem is not how to believe me, but in the emitting and reinforcement of new behavior of being assertive and making trouble.)

CASE ILLUSTRATION

Gary came into therapy with the first author because of a history of personal relationships that began well but subsequently became superficial and unsatisfying, ending because of "bad" feelings that developed. In addition, he had a long-standing problem of depression that seemed to vary with the quality of current interpersonal relationships. He was now in an important relationship with a woman which appeared to be following the ill-fated course of previous ones.

Gary seemed to be warm and likable, and did not appear to have any difficulty in relating to me during the early stages of therapy. Starting with history taking, treatment included directive approaches involving rational emotive therapy, behavioral rehearsal, and couples therapy. The original therapy contract of 10 sessions was extended to 20 sessions over a 9-month period. During this first phase of therapy, discussions of Gary's problem centered on behavior occurring outside the session in the recent and distant past. The early childhood origins of his problem were also explored. These discussions helped him to piece together a reasonably plausible verbal repertoire corresponding to the relationship between his history and the currently operating controlling variables that related to his presenting problem.

Thus, at the end of the 20 sessions, Gary had learned that his relationships seemed to sour when he got angry or irritated at his partner without discussing his concerns with her. He would become increasingly depressed, his partner would respond in kind with depression or anger, and eventually they would split up. During the initial course of treatment, Gary had agreed to express his negative feelings to his woman friend. He made this agreement because he felt that not doing so led to a lack of openness, lingering bad feelings, and eventual deterioration of the relationship. Even though Gary had this awareness of the problem, and had gone through cognitive therapy, behavioral rehearsal, and conjoint therapy aimed at helping him with the problem behavior, he still did not adequately express negative feelings and the relationship ended as had previous ones.

With each successive session following the breakup, Gary grew more reticent and depressed. When asked about his growing depression, Gary's interpretation was that it was due to mourning over the lost relationship and his inadequacy. I also observed within-session increases in the severity of his depression and therefore shifted the focus of treatment to this depression, the negative self-thoughts and the loss of hope that he would ever have a successful relationship.

With the application of Rule 1, I hypothesized that Gary's problems were being manifested in the session. When Gary was asked if he were angry with me or had other negative feelings, he denied that any were present or that his reticence or depression had anything to do with me. Although not completely convinced, I dropped the topic of the client-therapist relationship for the moment and concentrated on behavior therapy for depression. I became increasingly uncomfortable during the sessions, however, and found it difficult to keep the interaction going. For his part, Gary seemed to become even more depressed. When I suggested that Gary see a physician to try some antidepressant medication, he exploded in a tirade about M.D.s' not knowing what they are doing and causing more harm than good.

Hypothesizing that Gary's comments about M.D.s was stimulated by his reaction to me (see Chapter 3, Multiple Causation), I made this behavioral interpretation (Rule 5):

T: It looks like it's happening now—your problem that is. Our relationship started out fine, it started out very relaxed and open. You had no trouble in telling me about all your feelings and problems, and I looked forward to our sessions. The way our therapy started sounds like the way most of your past relationships started. Then things started going bad. You couldn't voice your negative feelings to Joyce even though we tried a variety of therapeutic approaches. Your relationship ended. You started getting depressed and became less open in our sessions. This gradually worsened to the present point—you have very little to say and I am finding the sessions frustrating because I don't know what to do that might help.

C: It feels the same as times in the past. And I have been thinking about quitting. (Adds to evidence that CRB1 is occurring.)

T: So our relationship is even headed for the final step that seems to have occurred so often in the past; it will end on a sour note. (For a comparison between within-session and daily-life behavior see Chapter 3.)

C: And I feel depressed and lousy about it. This is what always happens and I feel frustrated too because I don't know what to do.

T: Well, now you have a chance to make our relationship different and not feel lousy or frustrated. You can either let our relationship end like the others and you will continue to be unhappy and depressed, or you can be different and maybe feel better.

C: What do you mean be different—I don't know what to do.

T: Based on your past pattern, there must be negative and/or angry feelings toward me.

C: All I know is that I'm depressed and I want some help because it feels lousy. (CRB1-avoidance.)

T: You didn't answer my question. I said that I thought you had negative or angry feelings toward me. (Rule 3, blocking avoidance.)

C: I don't, can't we get back to my depression. (CRB1, avoidance.)

T: I think you are avoiding something about me that bothers you. When you first started therapy, I said I would try to help. Right now you are asking for help and I am trying to direct you to a topic that you don't think is related and you try to change the topic. (Rule 2, presenting the evocative situation—I am again trying to help right now, which has not worked previously; the failure of my previous interventions to help is hypothesized to evoke Gary's negative feelings and subsequent avoidance. Rule 3, blocking avoidance, and Rule 5, a behavioral interpretation, also are demonstrated here.)

C: I did everything you asked me to do and Joyce still left me. (CRB2)

T: You did what I asked and Joyce still left you and . . .

C: And you didn't help like you said you would. (CRB2, the first complaint ever directly expressed to me)

T: I tried, but it didn't come out well, and you did do everything that I asked. I feel bad about that and wonder what I should have done differently so that Joyce and you could have stayed together. I think it's important that you brought it up, and I want to see what can be done at this time. (Rule 3 is being followed; that is, the natural reinforcement for a complaint is to take it seriously and try to do something about it. In subsequent sessions, I observed in Gary an increase in expressions of dissatisfaction with therapy and with me, Rule 4.)

The therapeutic relationship intensified after this point, with more and more open expressions of emotional reactions between Gary and me. As the sessions almost exclusively focused on our relationship, Gary went into more detail about his disappointment in me and related issues of trust. Positive feelings of caring and warmth were also expressed. The original CRB1s of avoidance appeared less frequently, but whenever I detected one, I blocked it and an opportunity was provided for the development of Gary's new repertoire of open expression of negative feelings involving trust, disappointment, and anger. Gary became skilled at noting clinically relevant behavior as they occurred (CRB3), which, in turn, led to an even better therapeutic relationship. The repertoires developed in therapy readily transferred to the outside environment, and Gary reports that he is in the most satisfying intimate relationship he has ever had.

3

Supplementation

Enhancing Therapist Awareness of Clinically Relevant Behavior

Therapeutic helpfulness comes from noticing client behaviors that are instances of clinically relevant behavior (CRB). We have observed that the more CRBs that are detected, the more profound, intense, emotional, and fascinating the therapy. Any method or concept that can help in CRB detection thus has a place in FAP, especially because occurrences of CRB during the session are not always easily noticed. Since CRBs are weak variables controlling the therapist's observations, they usually require supplementation (Skinner, 1957) in order to increase their control. In the following sections (Classification of Verbal Behavior and Therapeutic Situations That Evoke CRB) our aim is to provide supplementation for increasing therapist skill or competence in observing CRB, sometimes called *sensitivity* or *insightfulness*.

CLASSIFICATION OF VERBAL BEHAVIOR

In any human endeavor, a classification system or taxonomy stimulates closer observation. For example, a little girl who learns to classify insects will look for and see more bugs, and when she finds one, she will be sure to notice the number of legs. Thus, we propose a classification system that enhances observation of CRB. The classification of verbal behavior helps increase therapist competence in observing CRB in two ways. First, it describes the type of client statements that lead to

47

CRB detection. Second, it capitalizes on the notion that each time your client makes a statement, it is possible that CRB has occurred—even though it may not appear so at face value.

The following example illustrates how using our classification system can lead to productive therapeutic intervention. A session with Karen, who was treated by the first author, began with:

T: How was your week?

C: Last week was really rotten, I got a $108 ticket [*sigh*] for expired license tags.

Our verbal classification system led me to consider that there was more to Karen's response than meets the eye. Given my knowledge of Karen, several possibilities occurred to me:

1. In receiving the ticket, she was caught at a wrongdoing; perhaps that's how she views therapy and thus reacts to me as she does to a policeman.
2. Perhaps she is concerned about the cost of therapy and paying for her bill.
3. She is obviously upset about the ticket and perhaps her comment really meant "please help me feel better."
4. She may have brought up this problem because she did not do the homework assignment I gave her, and bringing up the ticket was a way to evoke sympathy or direct attention away from the feared topic.
5. Perhaps she saw a policeman just before the session or noticed an airplane ticket lying on the receptionist's desk as she passed by.

I then proceeded to check out some of these hypotheses, and here is what happened when I asked about the bill:

T: What about our bill, are you worried about that?

C: No, because my insurance has a $100 deductible, and I've used over that in drugs already. So that covers my deductible and they've assured me that the first ten visits would be covered. I don't know about after that but they've been really good.

T: The reason I'm bringing up my bill is I'm trying to find out what would bother you about owing me money.

C: I don't like owing anybody money.

T: I know, but let's get down to real specifics. What would bother you?

C: I think about it a lot, and dollar signs ring every time I walk in the door.

The last statement supported the hypothesis that Karen's concern about fees manifested itself in her comments about the ticket incident. More importantly, however, my hypothesizing about "hidden" meanings led me to discover that Karen worried about owing me money in much the same way she worried about owing others money. Her worrying and anxiety about numerous unpaid bills was the focus of cognitive restructuring therapy in previous sessions, and she had avoided further work on this topic by reporting that it was no longer a problem. As the transcript indicates, it still was a problem. Her lack of awareness and indirect way of dealing with this problem during the session, however, resembled the inadequate approach she used during daily life. The identification of this CRB1 alerted me to the therapeutic opening. Here was an *in vivo* opportunity to block Karen's avoidance and encourage more adaptive ways of resolving the problem. During the next 6 months, Karen developed better repertoires for dealing with unpaid bills through learning how to deal with my unpaid bill. It also led to therapeutic work on a more general problem concerning her responses to others when she felt she was being negatively evaluated.

Some of our readers may wonder if our speculating about hidden meaning is within the realm of behaviorism, and furthermore, may think that it sounds suspiciously similar to psychoanalysis. Later, when we explain our verbal behavior classification system, we will show how radical behavioral theory leads to this type of interpretive activity. But for now, the radical behaviorist's inclusion of hidden meanings will be illustrated by the story about the friendly challenge to behaviorism by Alfred North Whitehead. While dining with Skinner in 1934, Whitehead said to him, "Let me see you account for my behavior as I sit here saying 'no black scorpion is falling on this table.'" The very next morning, Skinner started writing *Verbal Behavior*—a behavioral account of language. In the epilogue of this book, which took 23 years to complete, Skinner drew upon behavioral principles to account for Whitehead's statement. One conclusion was that the meaning of Whitehead's "black scorpion" was behaviorism. Skinner's interpretation was derived from his contextual theory of meaning that forms the core of the behavioral approach to language. Since Skinner, an avowed behaviorist, used behavioral principles to discover a hidden meaning in a statement made some 23 years earlier, it seems fair to argue that such an endeavor is within the realm of behaviorism. In fact, the therapist is even in a better position than Skinner to make behaviorally based interpretations of client comments since (1) they can be made immediately after the comments occur, (2) the therapist is in close contact with the circumstances surrounding the statement, and (3) the therapist continues to interact with the client and can gather additional information on the validity of the interpretation.

Although the interpretive activity may sound like what a psychoanalyst does, profound differences exist in terms of underlying assumptions and clinical implications. First and foremost, the behavioral therapist must remain humble by keeping in mind that the interpretations are only hypotheses. Further, the validity of the interpretations are difficult to evaluate because the controlling variables cannot be isolated in a laboratory setting. Behavioral theory suggests that the hidden meanings (actually, hidden causes and controlling variables) are in the surrounding environment, are not necessarily clinically relevant, and are not the result of something within the person that is striving for expression. Our account of client verbal behavior suggests that psychoanalytic interpretations are useful when they lead the analyst to observe CRB. Since FAP is specifically designed to increase CRB observation, it accomplishes this task more efficiently.

The FAP Client Response Classification System

Client responses or verbal behavior can be cues to the therapist to use the FAP classification system in order to arrive at the possible causes of their behavior as it is occurring. The FAP classification system is based on concepts from Skinner's *Verbal Behavior* (1957). An often maligned* but rarely read book, it is a rich source of concepts that can help detect CRB in the psychotherapy setting. It is a difficult book to read and the concepts are not easy to understand. Since we have used some of Skinner's concepts, and although we have made an effort to make our classification understandable, it may be beyond the interest of many of our readers. So, those of you who are not interested in learning the classification system in detail at this point, go on to the next section, which summarizes its implications. Then, skip the details of classification and go ahead to the next section on Therapeutic Situations That Frequently Evoke CRB.

*Most notable is Chomsky's (1959) review, which has been accepted by many as the definitive critique that justly discredited *Verbal Behavior*. Much of Chomsky's review, however, is aimed at methodological behaviorism, which Skinner vehemently rejected and thus was not the approach used in *Verbal Behavior*.

Implications of the Response Classification System for Doing FAP

The suggestions given below foster the development of the client-therapist relationship and CRB as well as making these a focus of the therapeutic interaction.

1. *Encourage and reinforce client descriptions that are related to stimuli present in the therapy environment.* These include any comment or description about the therapist, the therapeutic relationship, feelings about therapy (effectiveness, fees, attributes, defects, etc.), past interchanges or other events that occurred in the session, how they felt about coming to the session, any feelings they experienced during the session, the comfort or discomfort of the chair or lights, and so forth. Examples of therapist questions and statements that promote such client descriptions include: "How do you feel about coming in today?" "How did you feel after our last session?" "How do you feel about therapy?" "How do you think I feel about you?" "What are you thinking about?" "I'm upset at your hostility toward me." "I am wondering whether you think we are making sufficient progress." "I am thinking about what happened last week in our session."

2. *Encourage comparisons controlled by events in the therapy and in daily life.* Examples of such client statements are: "The anxiety I feel now is similar to what I feel when talking to the board of directors." "You remind me of my father." "You are the same as everyone else—you can't be trusted." "This is the only place I feel safe."

Examples of therapist questions and interpretations which encourage such client comparison statements include: "Is what just happened the same thing that happens when you see your mother?" "How does the way you are feeling now compare to how you felt at work?" "Can you compare your feelings about me to other people you have felt close to?" "The way you clammed up just now when I told you I cared about you seems similar to how you describe yourself to act when other people express affection."

3. *Encourage direct requests, suggestions, and wishes.* Examples of such client responses are: "Please help me get over my anxiety," "I need more attention," "I don't want to try to remember my childhood," "Can you lower your fee?"

Therapists can encourage client requests by explicitly stating, "It is permissible and desirable for you to want and ask for things from me. I will take all your requests seriously although I may not be able to

directly do as you wish." Modeling such behavior for clients is also helpful. Examples are "I would like you to come on time." and "I want to
talk about the money you owe me."

4. _Use client descriptions of events in their lives as metaphors for events_
occurring in the session. According to _Verbal Behavior_ principles, any client
response can be multiply determined; that is, there could be hidden motives (less obvious controlling variables) of which the client is not aware.
We suggest that you hypothesize about what these events in the session
might be and whether they are clinically relevant. For example, a client
describes how incompetent his dentist is. The therapist can respond, "I'm
wondering if you are concerned about whether I know what I am doing,"
or if early in the course of treatment, "Do you think psychotherapists
know what they are doing?"

The therapist can also speculate as to whether the metaphor is more
than a mere description of events that occur in the session. It could be
a disguised request and the therapist can hypothesize about what hidden
reinforcers might be involved. For example, if the client describes how
miserable the week has gone and how unhappy he has been, this could
be taken as a covert request with hidden reinforcers of sympathy and
for the therapist to not demand too much during the session.

Hidden motives can also be ascribed to direct requests. For example,
the client's request to terminate therapy might be reinforced by avoidance of conflict about being sexually attracted to the therapist.

Classifying Verbal Behavior

Skinner's approach is like no other linguistic classification system
because it classifies what is said on the basis of causes rather than on
its form or phonetic makeup. Although there are many levels of causes,*
those we are referring to are simply the discriminative stimuli that occur
before the response and the contingent stimuli that occur after it. The
first group is emphasized in defining the "tact" and the latter for the
"mand." These two terms _tact_ and _mand_ play a central role in our classification system and refer to verbal behaviors that differ from each other
in their causes.

An overview of the classification process is depicted by the flowchart in Figure 1. The process starts with classifying the client response

*From a behavioral standpoint, there are (1) contingencies of survival causes (e.g.,
evolutionary or constitutional causes, (2) contingencies of cultural survival (e.g., the
practices of the culture), and (3) contingencies of reinforcement (Skinner, 1974).

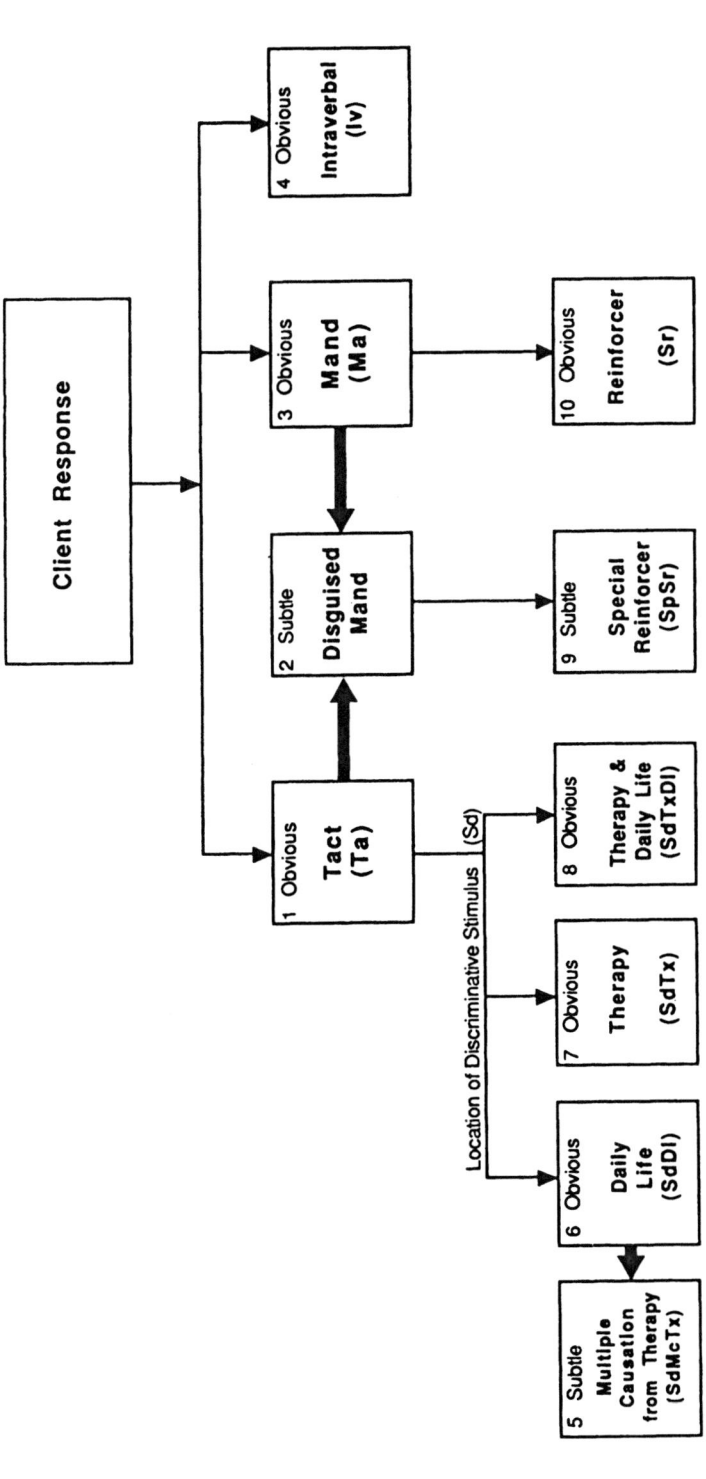

Figure 1. A classification of client statements. Bold arrows indicate points at which subtle interpretations are made.

as either a tact (Box 1), a mand (Box 3), or an intraverbal (Box 4). We view the classification system presented here as an introduction to using Skinner's verbal behavior principles in the psychotherapy setting. For pragmatic purposes, we have arbitrarily limited the number of verbal behavior concepts to the three mentioned above and do not exhaust the implications of the approach. Although a more complete application of verbal behavior would add even more to the therapeutic process, its discussion is beyond the scope of this book.

1. _The tact_. A *tact* is defined as a verbal response that is under the precise control of discriminative stimuli, and that is reinforced by generalized secondary reinforcers. For example, if you are shown a red ball and asked, "What is this?" and you say, "A red ball," you would be tacting because the form of your response ("red ball") is controlled by the object and is reinforced by a conditioned generalized reinforcer, such as "uh-huh," "right," or "thank you," or any of hundreds of reactions that indicate you were understood. Notice that the contingency or reinforcer is broad and general, whereas the prior discriminative stimulus (Sd) is specific.

The tact is thus brought about by the presence of a particular stimulus (e.g., a red ball) and an audience (the therapist or parent). Tacts, used in this sense, are similar to the notion of labels or names. However, since the terms *label* or *name* suggest the idea of symbolic representation, we use "tact" rather than "label" to underscore this difference. From a behavioral view, the words "red ball" do not symbolically represent or stand for the object any more than it could be said that a rat's lever press stands for or represents a yellow signal light in a Skinner box. The problem with a word "standing for" or "symbolizing" an object is that we now must explain what "standing for" or "symbolizing" means in order to understand the verbal response. Instead, by saying a tact is "controlled" by a prior discriminative stimulus, we can explain the behavior by referring to the well-understood process of discrimination. This process covers what others mean when they say a word is *symbolic* or stands for something. This does not mean, however, that we accept our clients' words at face value. Our position, illustrated in the $108 ticket example, leads us to quite the opposite view.

The location of the discriminative stimulus (Sd) that controls the tact is important in FAP verbal behavior classification. From our therapeutic viewpoint, the world can be divided into two types of Sds—those located in the therapy session or those in the client's daily life. The two types of Sds are shown in Figure 1, in Box 6 ($SdDl$) for daily life, and in Box 7 ($SdTx$) for therapy. A final category, reserved for those tacts that are evoked by *Sd*s located in both the client's therapy and in daily life, is shown in Box 8 (*SdTxDl*). So, if the "red ball" situation occurred during a therapy session, the tact "red ball" was brought about by an *SdTx* since the red ball was located in the therapy session.

A client describing a fight with her husband is emitting a tact under the control of a discriminative stimulus that is located in her daily life (e.g., an *SdDl* shown in Box 6). A client talking about a disagreement she had with her therapist is under the control of stimuli located in the therapy environment (e.g., an *SdTx* located in Box 7). The same client who says her fight with her husband is similar to her disagreement with the therapist is tacting under the control of stimuli located in the therapy and in daily life environments and is depicted in Box 8 (denoted as *SdTxDl*).

The primary focus of FAP is on responses that are controlled by stimuli occurring in the therapy session. Thus, the FAP therapist (1) is vigilant for and (2) encourages responses controlled by *SdTx* and *SdTxDl*. Identifying these responses, those controlled by *SdTx* and *SdDl*, clearly helps to determine which client responses are most important. For example, it points to the most important response among several emitted by Andrea, a client whose presenting problems are chronic unhappiness and social phobia. Here are her statements at the beginning of a session:

1. "Today I sort of lost my cool because I was called and told I had to be in Boise next week to interview for a secretarial job. And I don't know if I can do it, I don't know if I can go over there myself and go through with this."
2. "When I went out of here last week, I felt like skipping. I felt really good and I'm not sure why."
3. "I even had to schedule the interview so it wouldn't interfere with my taking medication. And that made me feel really foolish. I thought what if they knew about that, what if they knew that I couldn't come at noon because I had to get up in the middle and take a pill."
4. "If they knew that I was taking a tranquilizer, they wouldn't want to hire me."

These responses would all be classified as obvious tacts, but only one, Response 2, is controlled by a within-session stimulus—an *SdTx*. It is, therefore, the most clinically significant response (assuming that all are equally related to her presenting problems).

Keep in mind that a tact occurs merely because of the presence of the stimulus. This feature of the tact is particularly important in understanding the later discussion of multiple causation and so-called hidden meanings. We do not say that the client "uses" the tact to describe the stimulus any more than we would say that one "uses" a walk to get from here to there. We avoid viewing a client as "using" a verbal response because we are then faced with understanding what is being used. The "what" that is being used is the verbal response and we thus return to the original problem we are attempting to solve—that of understanding the verbal response. For example, let us say that you are attempting to arrive at the causes of a client's suicidal threats. If you were to say that the client "uses the threats," we then need to understand the causes of the behavior of "using" as well as the words being used. Instead, from our present perspective we would say the threat could be motivated by the attention they receive (a mand, as discussed below) or they could be controlled by presuicide behaviors (a tact) or some combination of the two. Furthermore, the client may or may not be aware of the controlling and/or motivating factors.

2. _The mand_. Mands are the speech involved in demands, commands, requests, and questions. A mand is behavior with the following characteristics: (1) it occurs because it was followed by a particular reinforcer, (2) its strength varies with the relevant deprivation or aversive stimulation, and (3) it appears under a very broad range of discriminative stimuli. Thus, if you were to say, "I would like some water" because you were thirsty, this would be a mand because it would be reinforced by a very specific reinforcer—someone hearing you and giving you water or showing you where to get some. Your "I want some water" response would not be reinforced by a generalized secondary reinforcer such as someone saying "That's right," or "Thanks for sharing that with me," or "I understand what you said." Its strength would also vary with how water deprived you were. Your mand for water can occur in almost any setting where you are thirsty and there is another person who can hear you.

Similarly, if a client were to say, "I want to have an extra session this week," it would be reinforced (and hence likely to occur again) by receiving an extra session (a specific reinforcer). The mand may indirectly involve deprivation or aversive states as in "Please take me for a ride," or "Don't abandon me." Behavior on the part of a client that occurs specifically because it evokes caring from the therapist is a mand.

As shown in Figure 1 and stated previously, the first classification called for is whether the client response is a tact (Box 1), a mand (Box 3), or an intraverbal (Box 4). The _intraverbal_ is verbal behavior evoked by verbal stimuli and generally covers those responses that cannot be classified as a tact or mand. For example, when asked "How are you," a response "Fine" usually is an intraverbal since it really does not have to do with the speaker's feelings but is simply an appropriate response to the string of words "how are you" (if "fine" really were based on the speaker's feelings, then it would be a tact and not an intraverbal). Client answers to such questions as "Where were your parents born?" and "Where does your partner work?" are intraverbals.

3. *Disguised mands.* You cannot be certain whether a given response is a tact or mand on the basis of its form (or sound). The word *fire*, for example, could be a mand to a firing squad or a tact under the control of a conflagration. Whereas classifying verbal behavior on the basis of its form or sound is called a *formal analysis*, Skinner's method of classifying on the basis of causes is called a *functional analysis*. Using Skinner's functional approach, the more we know about the context and history leading up to the response, the more certain we can be about its causes and its classification as a tact, a mand, or an intraverbal. Thus, if you see the conflagration and the speaker pointing at it, you have enough context to confidently classify the response as a tact.

The "fire" example illustrates that the same word can have different causes. The meaning of a word (or sentence, gesture, soliloquy, etc.) corresponds to its function, that is, a delineation of its causes. When we say the "same" word can have "different" meanings, "same" refers to the formal aspects of the word (the way it sounds and the way it is spelled) and "different" refers to its functional aspects. Consider the example of a client who says, "I am going to kill myself." If the client's response is primarily due to presuicide behaviors, such as suicidal plans and certain feelings that are associated with these, then the statement is a tact. If the statement is primarily maintained by concern that is evoked in others, then it is a mand. In our classification scheme, the former is shown as a tact in Box 1 and the latter is shown as a disguised mand in Box 2. It is a disguised mand because it looks like a tact based on its form, but in fact is a mand based on its function. Nonbehaviorists might prefer to differentiate the two suicidal statements on the basis of the client's intention or purpose. Although these terms convey a similar meaning, they can also be confusing and misleading. For example, does intention or purpose imply awareness and, if not, what does it mean to have an unconscious intention? Using our tact versus mand approach, awareness is a separate issue and has nothing to do with our classification. Thus, the client may or may not be aware of why he makes the suicide threat, and it can still be classified as to whether it is a tact or a mand. Further, if we do use intention or purpose to explain the client's suicide threat, the next step in therapy would be to discover where the intention or purpose came from. Tacts and mands, on the other hand, are already defined in terms of their origins.

The example of the suicide threats showed how the same utterance can have different meanings. Correspondingly, different utterances, such as "Please love me" and "I'm worthless and despicable" can have the same meaning (causes). The direct request for love may be caused by a past history of getting love and care when solicited and/or the present lack of love and care.* Because the form and function are consistent, we would say that this client means what he or she says. The response falls into Box 3 and is abbreviated as *Ma*. The reinforcer for this mand, loving care, enters into the classification system as shown in Box 10 and is represented as *Sr*. The latter statement about being worthless could also be caused by a desire for love and caring. Thus, it is a mand even though it sounds like a tact; that is, in this client's life experience, love and caring were more likely to occur after self-derision and not after a direct request. As pointed out earlier, these mands in tacts' clothing are referred to as *disguised mands* (Box 2). The reinforcer that is contingent on disguised mands are referred to as a special reinforcer, *SpSr* (Box 9), in order to signify that a specific reinforcer appropriate to a mand is involved and not merely the generalized secondary reinforcement that is contingent for tacts.

Thus, it is possible to have statements that are formally similar and yet are functionally different (the suicide example) as well as formally different yet functionally similar (the love and caring example).

4. *Multiple causation and supplementary stimulation.* Most verbal behavior is multiply determined. In addition to a primary controlling stimulus, there are usually additional supplementary controlling stimuli that also influence the response. This is obvious in slips of the tongue where the multiple causes produce a distorted response. The woman who tells her boyfriend that she will meet him for dinner at *sex* o'clock is an example. The response "sex" is a result of the simultaneous presence of primary stimuli evoking the response "six" and supplementary ones evoking "sex" although the ones for sex are less apparent to an outside observer. Most multiple causation, however, is less dramatic and does not produce an obviously distorted response. Instead, it may account for why a particular comment is being made at this time when

*One circumstance would be that the client has a history of never getting anything from others unless it was asked for directly and forcefully. Thus, although love and caring may not have been there, the mand occurs now because of the high strength of manding in general.

many others are also possible. A female client who is being supplementarily stimulated by her worries about the harmful effects of therapy may talk about her experience in the preceding week with an incompetent chiropractor. Another client who is supplementarily stimulated by his anger at the therapist might bring up an incident in which he lost his temper at his partner. Skinner refers to this process as *response selection* and proposes it as an alternative to saying the client has "chosen" the particular utterance from among those available.

Multiple causation, disguised mands, and special reinforcers are concepts that explain what traditionally have been referred to as _hidden, latent, or unconscious_ meanings. Consequently, we have thus given a behavioral account of such phenomena as slips of the tongue and how clients can say one thing but mean another. Clients are usually not aware of these variables, but they have their effects independent of awareness. We do not account for these effects by positing an inner mechanism, such as the unconscious. Instead, we refer to them as effects of *subtle* variables. In contrast, *obvious* variables are those that formally correspond to the form of the response. A *metaphor*, as used in this book, refers to responses controlled by subtle variables. For example, a bad dental experience is the obvious variable that controls the client telling the therapist "My dentist hurt me." If the client is telling the therapist about the dentist at that particular time because he has also been hurt by the therapist, then the subtle variable is the hurtful experience with the therapist. According to our definition, the "my dentist hurt me" is a metaphor because it is a multiply caused response under partial control of a subtle variable. The client need not (and probably is not) aware that the subtle variable has affected what he said.

As shown in Figure 1, all client responses are first classified on the basis of obvious variables as being either a Tact (Box 1), a Mand (Box 3), or an Intraverbal (Box 4). Then, at those points indicated by the heavy black arrow (Boxes 1, 3, and 6), it is suggested that subtle variables be considered. For example, if on the basis of form, you have classified the response as an obvious tact (Box 1), and the location of the controlling stimuli is in daily life (Box 6), then speculate as to which subtle stimuli present in the session (Box 5) could have supplemented the obvious ones to make that response occur. For example, if the client is talking about a relationship with a friend, what elements in the therapy relationship are in common with the outside relationship that may be responsible for the client's bringing it up at this time? If the client describes his feelings about someone else, hypothesize that there is a similarity in feelings about you. If the client describes an event during the week, what could the therapy relationship have in common with that event?

Using the FAP classification system will help you to generate hypotheses about the subtle variables that might be influencing the client's comments. Once the hypothesis is made, further information can be collected to help confirm or reject it.

Classification and the Observation of Clinically Relevant Behavior

Here are some ways in which classification can help identify clinically relevant behaviors (CRBs) in your clients:

1. Some clients rarely or never observe themselves or others in the "here and now." The absence of here and now observations could be a CRB1 that interferes with intimate relationships. Here and now observation of self and others is derived from the response class of tacting controlled by events in the session—*TaSdTx* (Box 7). The principal method used to identify CRB1 is to ask clients to compare their in-session behavior to daily life (e.g., "You looked away and didn't say anything when I asked you to talk about your feelings toward me. Is this what happens with your partner?"). The client's comparison response would be a *TaSdTxDl* (Box 8).

2. *TaSdTxDl* (Box 8) responses also enter into the strengthening of CRB3, clients' descriptions of their behavior and its causes. CRB3 is a specialized form of a tact that is controlled by stimuli occurring during the therapy session. The shaping of CRB3 begins with the therapist's encouraging any tacts controlled by discriminative stimuli in the therapy (*TaSdTx*) and in both therapy and daily life (*TaSdTxDl*). A comparison of behavior in session versus in daily life enters into CRB3s that can help in the transfer of therapeutic gains to daily life.

3. Subtle responses often constitute CRB1s. First, they show a lack of awareness. Thus, when a subtle response occurs, it provides a therapeutic opportunity to increase awareness by prompting and reinforcing the appropriate CRB3. For example, if a male client is under the control of the subtle variable of being hurt by the therapist and tells the therapist about a painful dental experience, the client will benefit from being able to describe the subtle variable and how it affects him (CRB3). That is, the therapist should help the client to become aware of the variables affecting his behavior (Rule 5). We believe this behavioral process is very similar to what psychoanalysts describe as "making conscious the unconscious." Second, the reason that many controlling variables "go underground" and become subtle in the first place is probably due to the effects of aversive conditioning and thus indicates a CRB1 of avoidance.

Third, disguised mands are often CRB1s because they are indirect ways of asking for something and the direct approach is usually more effective.

4. Classifying client responses brings the therapist into better contact with the overall context of the client's behavior. Rather than taking the client's comments at face value, the classification system can help the therapist to see the response as the result of obvious and subtle variables that reflect the history of the client as well as the effects of the client-therapist relationship. Seeing the "bigger picture" increases sensitivity to CRB and the role of within-session reinforcement.

It is important to keep in mind that classification is not the only point at which CRB is considered during the therapy session. All client behavior should constantly be evaluated for its CRB possibilities. A CRB evaluation is done even before the response is classified the bottom of the flowchart is reached. Consider, for example, a timid fearful client who never confronts those in authority who suddenly blurts out "You aren't paying attention to what I'm saying and this really irritates me." This immediately could be recognized as CRB2 and CRB3 without going through the verbal behavior classification process. The purpose of the classification process is to make visible more CRB than might be immediately detected but should not be seen as the only method for arriving at CRB. Let us now turn to the some examples of classification.

Examples of Classifications of Client Responses

1. *"It's ten to five, so it's time to leave."* According to the flowchart, we first ask, "Is this an obvious tact (Box 1), mand (Box 3), or intraverbal (Box 4)?" Our answer is "obvious tact" since the clock apparently is the controlling stimulus accounting for the specific form of the response "ten to five" which, in turn, serves as a cue for the end of the session. As we proceed in the flowchart, we determine the discriminative stimulus (*Sd*) location. Since the client referred to the clock and it is located in the therapy session, it is an obvious *SdTx* (Box 7).

Now to the CRB evaluation: If a daily life problem of the client is that he compulsively lives by the clock and "must" end exactly on time, the response is a CRB1. However, if the client's comment is an improvement over his typical time compulsiveness seen in previous therapy sessions (just getting up and leaving), the response is a CRB2. The flowchart also directs our attention to subtle factors; that is, the possibility that the response might be a disguised mand (Box 2).

For example, a female client might want you to stop asking questions about her feelings. The special reinforcement would then be the avoidance of further discussion of the topic at hand. Since this is a subtle interpretation, the indirect nature of the response could be a CRB1.

2. *"My wife refused to do the laundry."* Again, we first ask, "Is this an obvious tact, mand, or intraverbal?" It is a tact, Box 1, assuming that the actual event of the wife refusing to do the laundry is the controlling variable for the response. The location of this event is the client's daily life (*SdDl* Box 6). In evaluating CRB possibilities, if the client previously had been fearful of being critical of his wife, then this would be a CRB2. Next, as indicated on the flowchart, a subtle interpretation of a disguised mand (Box 2) is called for. It is possible that the client is not merely "reporting the facts" as implied by the obvious tact but instead (or in addition) has hidden motives (e.g., subtle, special reinforcers [Box 9]). Possible special reinforcers are that the client wants the therapist to say something like "What an irresponsible wife you have," "Here is how to make your wife do the laundry," or "That's too bad, at a time you're already so stressed out." A possible CRB1 related to the hidden motivations would be "wanting others to be supportive of him in his marital and other interpersonal conflicts but not asking for this directly."

3. *"How much do you charge per session?"* The response is an obvious mand (Box 3) because it specifies a specific reinforcer (Box 10). The obvious reinforcer is the therapist stating the fee. It is possible that the mand is not as it appears and instead involves a subtle, special reinforcer, *SpSr* (Box 9). The most obvious of these concerns the amount charged by the therapist. For example, the client could mean "Lower your fee." This hidden motivation would indicate the CRB1 of not being direct or not being aware. If the client avoided making commitments in general, then another CRB1 could be the avoidance of making a commitment to start therapy by using the fee as an excuse.

4. *"Nobody likes me."* Based on its form, the response is an obvious tact (Box 1). The location of the controlling *Sd* appears to be an *SdTxDl* (Box 8) because "nobody" could also refer to the therapist. If the client's presenting problem, in her words, is that "she is unlovable," then the response indicates that CRB1 is occurring. In terms of a subtle interpretation, the disguised mand (Box 2) could be "Please, like me" or "Tell me that you like me." The indirect or unaware quality of the disguised mand could be a CRB1.

5. *"I feel nauseated."* This is an obvious tact (Box 1) because the response appears to be controlled by stimulation from the stomach. The

location of the Sd controlling this tact is in the therapy session, an *SdTx* (Box 7). In general, feeling statements are obvious tacts because they are taken to be controlled by prior stimuli. It is of incidental interest that the controlling stimuli are private. The response indicates that a CRB1 is occurring if nausea is a presenting problem or a CRB2 if the client never complains about physical problems. A subtle interpretation is that the response is a disguised mand for empathy or avoidance of what was happening before the complaint was made.

THERAPEUTIC SITUATIONS THAT FREQUENTLY EVOKE CLINICALLY RELEVANT BEHAVIOR

There are stimuli common to the therapeutic situation that often precipitate client behavior that may be clinically relevant. We are calling attention to these situations with the hope that they will be observed as they occur during the session.

1. *Time structure*. Therapy hours are scheduled to start and end at a certain time. The client may come late, give excessive attention to arriving early, wish to leave early, or not leave on time. Coming late to an appointment can be related to presenting problems, such as the avoidance of emotionally laden discussions, the planning of time, or work problems produced by not being punctual. Having difficulty in leaving at the end of the hour can be related to behavior, such as excessive dependence or clinginess that has caused problems in other relationships. Inordinate attention paid to promptness can be related to such presenting problems as compulsiveness or extreme fear of disappointing others associated with a lack of self-worth.

Coming late to appointments when therapeutic progress is occurring also may be an instance of the presenting problem for the client who has difficulty in completing tasks and who seems to "screw up" situations in which he or she could be successful. Coming late or leaving early can be instances of clinically relevant operants for a client who presents anxiety problems. In each case, the operant behavior observed during the session is evaluated for possible relevance to the particular client's presenting problems.

2. *Therapist vacations*. Some clients, especially those with histories of rejection and abandonment, react strongly to disruptions in the pattern of contact with the therapist. For these clients, the therapist's going away

can elicit intense fear, anxiety, anger, and/or sadness with accompanying thoughts such as "You won't come back," "You're trying to get away from me because I was 'bad'," "You'll be different and won't care about me when you get back," "How can you leave me right now when I need you so much?" "I can't live without you," and "I can't take care of myself." Most behavior that accompanies such feelings (other than talking about them) are CRB1 (e.g., becoming withdrawn, breaking things, attempting suicide).

3. *Termination.* The most difficult type of termination is the ending of an incomplete treatment because of factors in the therapist's life, such as changing jobs, moving, or ending an internship. This can bring forth the feelings described under 2 in an even more intensified fashion. In mutually agreed upon terminations, it is a time for the therapist to be vigilant for CRB evoked by endings. Terminations can bring up concerns about self-reliance and independence, and grief about previous losses, separations, and deaths. It is a chance for the client to learn to say good-bye properly by expressing the range of feelings engendered by the ending of a special, but transitional relationship. How the client reacts to termination is likely to be an indication of how he or she reacts to endings and beginnings in other areas of life.

4. *Fees.* How a client handles therapy fees can be representative of the way he or she deals with money elsewhere. Does the client pay on time? Does the client manage bills and budgeting poorly? The fee issue can be brought into the treatment in numerous ways: (a) It can lead to termination and withdrawal behaviors that are associated with statements like "I don't deserve to be spending this money on me, other family members are more important and deserving of funds than me." (b) It can be used to avoid feelings of closeness toward the therapist— "You're being nice to me because I pay you and that's your job." (c) It can be used to explore the behavior and/or affect evoked by making (or not making) a certain amount of money; feelings of success, inferiority, incompetence, insecurity, shame; competitiveness with or envy toward the therapist. (d) Rather than directly expressing negative feelings to the therapist about fees, avoidance may involve the client's being late with payments. (e) The client may try to get the therapist to lower the fee by understating the amount of money earned. (f) If the client is in a financial crisis, can he or she accept the idea of carrying a balance, in essence, taking a loan from the therapist? Critical behaviors involving giving and taking in relationships, and not wanting to owe anybody

anything, to the point of one's detriment, are often observed at these times.

5. *"Mistakes" or unintentional therapist behavior*. The saying "It's grist for the therapy mill" applies here. The best of therapists may come late to the session, run overtime with the previous client, lapse into day-dreams while the client is talking about something important, forget to make a phone call he promised the client he would make, or otherwise act in ways that result in the client's feeling unimportant or misunder-stood. How does your client react to a less than perfect therapist? Thera-pist errors are occasions in which CRBs such as these can be evoked: avoidance of direct expression of anger and frustration, problems asso-ciated with feelings of lack of worth to oneself and to significant others, or extreme reactions to therapist mistakes associated with idealizing oth-ers so much that disillusionments are inevitable. Any of these behaviors can interfere with the development of a stable relationship.

6. *Silences and lapses in the conversation*. The most salient feature of adult psychotherapy is that it consists of two people talking to each other. It is common for this conversation to run into dead ends and stop—both people seem to have nothing to say. This situation can evoke CRB in the client, not to mention the therapist. A lapse in the conver-sation evokes anxiety and accompanying confusion which in turn makes it even more difficult to start talking again. The anxiety, confusion, and difficulty in resuming the interaction are the problem. Learning to tol-erate the silences more, extinguish anxiety, and/or develop stronger con-versation-resuming behavior at the time that conversation stalls would constitute CRB2.

7. *Expression of affect*. We are referring to the showing of feelings that results from contact with stimuli eliciting those respondents called *emotions* and/or *describing feelings*. Our view of emotions is given in Chapter 4, which provides a more complete explanation and provides the rationale for our comments in this section. Expression of affect, such as sadness, need, vulnerability, anger, and caring, facilitates the devel-opment and maintenance of close relationships. There are, however, many factors that hinder the expression of affect. Thus, for example, many clients have trouble crying in front of others and expressing anger appropriately. Their discomfort with showing strong affect often hinders treatment. Clients have said that showing their feelings would mean "be-ing weak," "being one down," "being too vulnerable," "not being able to stop," "being out of control" or "being laughed at." Avoidance be-

haviors associated with showing affect include: changing the subject; talking endlessly in great detail about tangential topics; not talking; focusing on an object in the office; counting backward from 1,000 to oneself. In rare instances, the CRB is the client's deliberate use of anger or tears to control the behavior of others.

8. *Feeling good, doing well.* For some clients, feeling good or doing well serves as an aversive stimulus. This then motivates avoidance behavior in the form of being and acting miserable and depressed. Clients report feeling afraid, anxious, out of control, and that they are "waiting for the other shoe to drop." Their histories reveal experiences in which they had been punished in some way for feeling good, thereby giving "doing well" its aversive controlling properties. For example, a jealous and psychologically disturbed parent might withdraw or otherwise punish a child for being successful. Doing well might also signal losing the therapist because therapy will have to end. Needless to say, CRB1 consisting of depression and misery as avoidance of doing well or termination of treatment would seriously compromise long-term positive reinforcement for the client.

9. *Positive feedback and expressions of caring by the therapist.* Some clients do not react well to positive expressions by the therapist. The positive feedback may be reacted to as an arbitrary reinforcer, as a signal for increasing demands, or as a prelude to withdrawal of positive reinforcement. Clients may then resist, avoid, ignore or otherwise discount what the therapist has said. Their reactions also may be accompanied by feelings of embarrassment, unworthiness, discomfort, and such thoughts as "Now I'm going to have to live up to these expectations or you'll withdraw approval." "You don't really know me, and when you do, you'll leave." "You're just saying that to be nice and I don't believe you." All of these reactions can be acquired in families in which positive feedback has been associated with aversive consequences.

10. *Feeling close to the therapist.* When the therapist shows caring, concern, and understanding, or staying with the client through rough times, the client may feel close to the therapist. Such feelings normally accompany repertoires of maintaining contact which can include: spending more time with the person, physical closeness or contact; expressing positive feelings; doing things to help or protect the person. However, these behavioral repertoires may have been punished in the past by loss, rejection, or abandonment. Further, the limitations of the therapeutic relationship (time limits, contact restricted to the session, etc.) also result

in punishment of the "closeness repertoires." Whatever the causes, closeness is often an aversive *Sd* which motivates client behavior to remove it. Since this avoidance can be difficult to detect because many of the closeness behaviors cannot occur in the session, the therapist relies on the collateral feelings as a guide. When you are feeling close to the client, does she act in a way that facilitates closeness, or does she engage in behavior that decreases your feelings of closeness? A variety of avoidance reactions can result in distance, including becoming critical, getting angry, getting numb inside and not feeling anything, saying she doesn't need to come in anymore, or making comments that devalue the meaning of the relationship because it is a professional one. A primary step in remediation involves the client's learning to talk about the functional relationships (CRB3s), as in "I'm feeling close to you right now and I feel like staying with you and know I can't. This upsets me, so I want to distance you."

11. *Therapist characteristics*. Stable characteristics of the therapist, such as age, gender, race, weight, physical attractiveness, and behavioral tendencies to be talkative or quiet, gentle or confronting, self-disclosing or private, open-minded or opinionated, can evoke CRB. For example, an older male figure can be reminiscent of father; a confronting or talkative therapist can evoke unassertiveness accompanied by feelings of intimidation and powerlessness; a thin therapist can bring forth envy, withdrawal, and comments such as "There's no way you'll understand my problem" in an overweight client. Every therapist should try to get an idea of what their stable characteristics are and look for possible evocative effects of CRB.

12. *Unusual events*. Sometimes the most important CRB can occur under less common conditions. Examples of these idiosyncratic events include seeing the therapist with a partner outside of therapy; the therapist's becoming pregnant, breaking a leg, or leaving town for a family emergency can serve as powerful aversive stimuli that provoke behaviors such as intense feelings associated with possessiveness, sibling rivalry, dependence, helplessness, and mortality.

13. *Feelings or private states of the therapist*. The therapist's private reactions to the client can be a good source of information about clinically relevant behavior. Feelings of boredom, irritation, or anger in the therapist may indicate that the client is behaving in ways that are likely to elicit the same feelings in other people.

For example, a female client complains that she has trouble making friends and does not know why. You notice that you easily become bored with her and your attention drifts because she tends to talk in a monotone about trivial details for minutes at a time without checking to see whether you are interested in what she is saying. Thus, self-observation can aid in the discrimination of these problem behaviors and also can be used to detect improvements (CRB2), such as talking in a more animated fashion, curtailing her verbosity, and asking questions.

In summary, the therapeutic situations that we have examined are representative of the many ways that stimuli associated with therapy can evoke client CRB. The verbal behavior classification system presented in the first section of this chapter can help to increase awareness of CRB by focusing the therapist's attention on the subtle causes of client verbalizations. Clients' observations of themselves in the here and now, and also their comparisons of events in therapy to daily life, are descriptions that can help generalize their gains from therapy.

4

The Role of Emotions and Memories in Behavior Change

Emotions and memories have always occupied a central position in psychotherapy. Their utility is compelling, yet their definition and measurement are elusive. The radical behavioral foundations of functional analytic psychotherapy (FAP) bring a different perspective to these topics and to their relevance in clinical practice.

EMOTIONS

Many people wrongly accuse radical behaviorists of holding the black-box theory of emotion. According to this view, emotions occur inside the person (the black box), and therefore are outside the interest of the behavior analyst. As pointed out in Chapter 1, it is actually the methodological behaviorists who hold this view. In contrast, radical behaviorists think that "how people feel is often as important as what they do" (Skinner, 1989, p. 3).

In this chapter, the term *feeling* is used as a verb and as a noun. When used as a verb, feeling is an activity, a type of sensory action, such as seeing or hearing. When its function is a noun, feeling is used interchangeably with the terms *emotion* and *affect*. Just as there are objects that are seen, feeling as a noun is the object that is felt, as in "I feel a feeling." What is the object being felt, however, when we feel depressed? Other objects, like a frozen yogurt cone, can be seen, felt, and tasted; that is, the object (frozen yogurt cone) can be known in several ways. If we are not sure of what we are seeing, we can taste it or even ask someone else what it is. Such is not the case when the object is depression or anxiety—we can only feel it.

The behavioral view asserts that what we feel is our body. Of our three sensory nervous systems—*exteroceptive, interoceptive,* and *proprioceptive*—the latter two are involved in the feeling process. The proprioceptive nervous system carries stimulation from the muscles, joints, and tendons, and is involved with movement and posture. The interoceptive nervous system carries stimulation from the viscera, such as the bladder and the stomach, as well as from glands, ducts, and the vascular system. These two nervous systems are stimulated by the parts of the body involved in fear, anger, depression, anxiety, joy, and the like. Relatively little is known, however, about which particular organs are involved for the various feelings we experience. This paucity of knowledge is especially apparent when compared to what we know about the exteroceptive system. This third sensory nervous system is involved in seeing, hearing, smelling, and touching, and the specific sensory organs are clearly identified as the eye, ear, nose, and skin.

Up to this point we have discussed (1) the activity of feeling or sensing the emotion, and (2) the object that is felt—the body. The question we will now address is, "How does the body get in that particular state which is then felt?" Our answer presumes that the state of the body is "a collateral product of environmental causes" (Skinner, 1974, p. 242). Thus, for every behavior there is a corresponding bodily state. When engaged in the behavior we classify as talking, for example, the muscular-skeletal system and the nervous system are in a particular state that changes along with the words being spoken. When we say the word "hello," the many muscles required for this task are in a particular position, which then changes as we continue to say, "How are you?" Similarly, when we are engaged in the operant and respondent behaviors of being emotional, there are also states of the body that are correlates of those responses. For illustrative purposes, these bodily states may include changes in heart rate, pupil dilation, blood vessel constriction, glandular secretions, and muscle contractions. In actuality, the current state of knowledge precludes any precise physiological measurement of these states. All that is relevant to our discussion is that a person experiences different bodily states, known only to him or her, in correspondence with different emotions.

Emotional operant and respondent responses are evoked by particular situations. For example, Skinner (1953, p. 166) described a situation in which a man was criticized at work. This man reacted with an emotional response pattern that is called *anger*. This pattern included the following responses: (1) respondent behaviors—the man turned red, his hands sweat, he stopped digesting his lunch, his face took on the characteristic expression of anger (furrowed brow, flared nostrils, snarled lips), and (2) operant behaviors—he spoke curtly to his fellow workers, slammed a door, kicked a cat, and watched a street fight with special interest. There was a bodily state correlated with this pattern of operant and respondent responses. If the man engaged in the activity of feeling this bodily state, then he would *feel* angry. However, others who observed this person would say he *was* angry, even if the man did not feel the anger himself.

This description of the man's total response to criticism at work, including both his operant and respondent behaviors, is not intended to be a concise and complete description of anger. Instead, the description is simply this man's responses at the time, which are viewed by himself and others as anger. In general, the variety and nuances of emotions suggest that attempting to classify them definitively would be nearly impossible.

Sometimes clients will lament that they feel one way but act in another. This comment may not seem to make sense from a behavioral standpoint since all that can be felt are bodily states that are collaterals of actions (responses). Thus, the client has two bodily states that can be felt, but only says that one of them is a feeling. A behavioral interpretation of this comment is that bodily states associated with respondents are experienced more intensely than bodily states associated with operants. Often operant behavior affects respondent behavior, but when it does not, the result is feeling one way and acting another. For example, suppose the angry man in the foregoing example behaved in all the ways described except that he petted the cat and forced a friendly smile. Now if he said he *acted* friendly but *felt* angry, the feeling he referred to would be of the bodily states associated with anger, but not the bodily states associated with smiling and petting the cat. If we can assume that he really does feel the bodily collaterals of petting and smiling as well as the other responses, it would be more accurate for him to say, "I feel two ways and they are different but one of the ways I feel (collaterals of smiling and petting) is not my true feeling." The basis of these two different kinds of feelings has to do with the reasons for his petting the cat and smiling. In particular, he might be aware that the petting and the smiling are the result of social contingencies to make him "be calm and civil." He does not view the feelings associated with behavior caused by such contingencies as relevant to his true feelings.

As outlined below, clinical problems sometimes involve the opposite scenario; that is, the feeling or sensing of public responses under control are what the client reports to be the true feeling and the private responses are not noticed (e.g., the man would report feeling affectionately toward the cat and not notice his anger feelings). In this case, the client is described as not being in touch with his feelings, and the therapist's task is to shift the control to those bodily states that are more private.

Learning the Meanings of Feelings

Of greater relevance to the psychotherapist than the activity of feeling is the process by which we learn what our feelings are. We are not born knowing what our emotions are any more than we are born knowing what a tree is. These must be taught by our parents. Since the object being felt is private, the parent who is trying to teach a child to identify (tact) feelings is at a disadvantage. In teaching the child to tact a public object like a tree, the parent can point to the tree, pronounce its name, and reinforce a response such as "ree." After several such experiences, the public stimulus, the tree, controls the response "tree." In the case of a feeling, the stimuli that we hope will gain control are private bodily states. In order to accomplish this, the parent must look at public stimuli, make a guess as to what is going on inside the child on the basis of these public stimuli, pronounce their names, and reinforce the appropriate response. For example, the parent may look at public stimuli, such as the time of day and the baby's crying, and guess that the private stimulus of hunger is present. The parent will then encourage the child to say "baby hungry." Eventually, if the parent were perceptive, the private stimulus of hunger would be tacted as "I'm hungry."

Such a learning process has several outcomes. First, the tacting and discrimination of feelings will not reach the reliability of tacting public objects, such as rocks and airplanes. Second, in the case of feelings, the public stimuli may inadvertently gain partial control of the tact because the parent cannot always be correct about which private feeling is present on the basis of public stimuli. For example, sometimes the parent will say "Baby is happy" on the basis of her smile, when the private stimulus is really only a gas pain. At other times, her smile is an accurate indication that private happiness is present and "baby is happy" is closer to the mark. As this child develops, the meaning of the word *happy* will depend on how often the private bodily states of happiness are present when she is prompted to say "happy." Instances in which this child is actually ill or in pain in outwardly "happy" situations (e.g., a birthday party) will interfere with her private bodily states' gaining control over her accurate tacting of feelings, unless someone notices and says, "Oh, you look sick." In essence, the meaning of happiness for this child is the outcome of discrimination training similar to that in concept-formation tasks. In these tasks, complex stimuli are presented in a series of trials (e.g., big blue circle, small blue circle; big red circle, small blue circle; big red triangle, small green triangle) where only certain aspects of the stimuli relevant to the concept (e.g., "bigger"). After a sufficient number of trials, these relevant aspects come to control the concept.

Since the parent uses public stimuli to identify the feeling to be tacted, the child may inadvertently come under partial control of these same stimuli. This phenomenon of inadvertent public control over a feeling is commonly recognized in the research literature on the control of hunger. Public stimuli, such as the time of day (lunchtime) and the attractiveness of the food, can result in "I'm hungry." As detailed in Chapter 6, it is not merely the verbal response that is controlled but the experience itself; that is, the person really experiences hunger as coming from within even when the response is largely controlled by the clock indicating noon and only minimally by a full stomach. An interesting implication of this view is that if it were possible for one person to feel another's feelings, they would be experienced as similar or different depending on the sources of control. Thus, if your hunger were controlled by private stimuli arising from your stomach, and you could feel another's hunger controlled by external stimuli, you would find these two experiences to be very different. The only feelings in common would be those associated with inclinations to eat and procure food.

Given the conditions under which tacting of feelings are acquired, any emotion could inadvertently come partially under public control, resulting in a confusion or mislabeling of actual internal experience.

Feelings as Causes of Behavior

An emotion or feeling is a state of the body. For every response there is an accompanying state of the body. For example, when running, an accompanying state of the body can be felt. Although both running and the collateral feelings are present, we usually do not say the running is caused by the feeling. Instead, we might say that we are running to catch the bus. That is, we do not attribute a causal role to feelings when, as in the case of running to catch a bus, a clear external cause can be identified.

There are other times, however, when clear external causes are not identified or known. For example, a woman who jogs daily might have forgotten or never have been aware of the external conditions (e.g., her best friend also doing it, her body being stronger, compliments from others about how good she looks) that brought her to the point of running every day. Under these conditions, we tend to attribute the cause to the collateral bodily state which is felt. Thus, the jogger might say she runs because she feels like it. Similarly, a person who is eating may say he is doing so because he was hungry. This usually means that the antecedents of both the collateral feeling of hunger as well as the eating are not identified and the feeling is given causal status.

Other situations also lead to causal attributions of feelings. Often, the feeling can be felt before the behavior is emitted. We can be hungry without eating, angry without being aggressive, and fearful without running away. In these cases, we have inclinations to act but do not. Since the action is absent or the feeling precedes the action, it is tempting to attribute causal status to the feeling.

The problem with attributing causal status to a collateral bodily state is that it may direct attention away from the factors that cause both the behavior (or inclination to act) as well as the collateral feeling.

For example, Jan, a client of the second author, who had trouble following through with the pursuit of her goals, attributed her lack of success to "a fatal character flaw, an inability to sustain myself." Dwelling on and trying to change these internal states that supposedly were responsible for her not finishing graduate school and vocational school only made Jan feel worse about herself and more helpless. I asked what had sustained her through six years of therapy with me, and she replied, "Different things at different times—my friends all being in therapy, habit, desperation, hope, a feeling of movement, my attachment to you, being validated by you." I suggested to her that one could not accomplish demanding tasks in a vacuum without external support, and that she had support from me and her friends which helped to sustain her through difficult times in therapy. In contrast, her parents had not been at all supportive of her choice of subject area in school, and she did not stay in school long enough to make friends there or to reap much in the way of rewarding experiences. By focusing on the external conditions leading to her successes and failures, and looking at the internal states or feelings as collaterals, Jan was more hopeful that she could change her behavior. Even though feelings may not cause behavior, as pointed out later, the expression of feelings does play an important role in FAP.

Hayes (1987) has based a therapeutic system on the problems caused by clients who view their feelings as causal. According to Hayes, the incorrect view of the causal nature of feelings leads clients to seek elimination of thoughts and feelings so as to change their behavior and have a better life. Efforts aimed at the elimination of feelings, however, are fundamentally faulty because the problem is not the feeling but instead the clients' efforts to change the feeling. Comprehensive distancing,

Hayes's therapeutic system, is an ingenious approach that uses metaphor and experiential methods to undermine the client's ineffective approach to solving problems.

Expressing Feelings

The expression of feelings refers to a continuum of behavior. One end of the continuum is referred to as *communicating feelings*. These are operant verbal behaviors whose purpose is to inform another about the speaker's feelings. "I feel angry" and "I love you" are examples. At the other end of the continuum are the showing of feelings—nonverbal respondent behaviors that are automatically elicited. These respondents would include blushing, laughter, primitive facial expressions, and sobbing. Located at different points on the continuum are responses that are partially respondent but that also have been shaped by contingencies. Examples are crying that has partially been shaped by the attention that it receives, the choking of words because of grief, the exclamation "ouch" which is elicited by a painful stimulus but which also shows the effects of contingencies (e.g., it is "ai-yoh" in Chinese).

Expressing feelings can be very useful in some situations, particularly in the development and maintenance of intimate relationships. Since difficulties in intimate relating are a common presenting problem, inadequate expression of feelings is frequently a focus of FAP. Intimate relationships by definition involve a sensitivity to the effects of one person's behavior on another. Prototypically, parents are quite aware of the reinforcing and punishing effects of their behavior on their infants. The parents' behavior, in turn, is shaped by the infant. This process occurs in part because parents are sensitive to the nuances of the infant's reactions. No matter how sensitive the parent is, however, intimacy can only occur if the infant expresses feelings. In the adult intimate relationship, expressing feelings plays the same role.

An expression of feelings also increases the likelihood that one's needs will be met (obtaining reinforcement from others). Needs can be met because an effective expression of feelings can evoke in the listener some of the same bodily states that are being expressed. This process is useful because listeners can then better predict the behavior of the communicator by asking themselves (1) how they would behave if they had the feelings just expressed, or (2) what kinds of behavior accompanied this person's expression of such feelings in the past. Knowing another person well, in turn, involves being able to predict what the other person will do (including predicting what would be reinforcing for that person). Intimate relationships seem to require a good deal of knowing what to expect from the other person and thus requires emotional expression.

Of the two types of emotional expression (communicating and showing), verbal statements (communicating) such as "I am happy" and "I feel sad" have the advantage of being easy to discriminate. The usefulness of simple tacts, however, is limited because the variety and nuances of feelings far exceed these simple one-word descriptions. Describing the state of the body is usually not as effective as describing analogies, metaphors, or external conditions that may bring about that feeling. The following are examples of such descriptions by our clients: (1) Feeling of not quite belonging—"It's like when you try to put a metric nut on a bolt of approximately the same size but the threads are SAE (a slightly different type of threading). It almost goes on and you keep on trying but it just doesn't fit." (2) Fear—"It's like I'm walking down a dark alley and I hear footsteps behind me, and I walk faster, and I hear the footsteps move faster." (3) Terror—"It's like I'm all alone in the house, and the electricity goes out. I can hear an intruder moving around in the basement, and I think he is trying to kill me. I pick up the phone to call for help and it is dead."

On the other hand, there are disadvantages to the use of communicating feelings as a means of emotional expression. The major one is that the meaning of the feeling may be highly idiosyncratic because of the ambiguity of controlling stimuli. One person's "I feel depressed" may have little in common with another's identical statement. A further disadvantage is that it is easy to mislead with verbal behavior. For example, "I love you" may be said just to get someone to have sex or to buy expensive presents. Also, the sensitivity of verbal behavior to social contingencies can easily result in saying what is socially appropriate rather than what one really feels.

The advantages of showing feelings (as opposed to communicating feelings) as a method of expressing feelings are that they are less subject to contingencies and thus are more spontaneous and less likely to mislead. For example, although it is possible to feign crying, it is relatively difficult to do convincingly. Similarly, it is almost impossible to stop a blush despite negative consequences. For most people, the range and nuances of the expressed emotions are greater with the showing of emotion than with verbal descriptions. It is for these reasons that the showing of feelings are particularly useful in FAP as indications of contact with important variables.

Avoiding Feelings

We have already discussed one of the causes for client difficulties in expressing feelings; that is, the client may not know how they feel because they never learned to come under the private control of their bodies. Diminished expression of feelings can also result from admonishment in numerous contexts. As children, expression of feelings might be punished by the parent because it is inconvenient or disruptive. Paradoxically, a major source of punishment is derived from one of the uses of the expression of feelings discussed in the previous section—expressing feelings allows others to know us and predict our behavior. Although such knowledge leads to positive reinforcement in an intimate relationship, it can also lead to punishment if the knowledge is used against us. Perhaps this is why emotional expression is sometimes described as "being vulnerable."

Expression of feelings is often punished in adult life because most cultures place substantial prohibitions on displays of emotion (Nichols & Efran, 1985). The reason for this cultural punishment is that the display means that the person is "off duty" and is not attending to the task at hand. This seems to hold true for a wide range of situations. A grocery clerk who emotionally responds because a customer reminds him of his abusive mother would suffer negative consequences, as would an airline pilot who "breaks down" in an emergency. It is often in the best interests of the culture to limit the expression of affect. The down side of limiting the expression of feelings is the problems it causes in relationships, particularly intimate ones.

When the expression of feelings is punished, the conditions that evoke the emotional responses also become aversive and are avoided. For example, if a child is punished for feeling and acting affectionate, then situations that evoke affection could also become aversive. Feeling affectionate (the bodily states associated with affection) might also be aversive because it is associated with punishment. It is important to note that the aversive feelings do not cause the avoidance of affection; the punishment caused this avoidance as well as the aversive feelings. To overcome this problem, one would not focus on the aversive feelings directly because they are simply a collateral state, but rather on the conditions that evoke the aversive feelings. Thus, the goal would be for the individual to no longer avoid conditions evoking affection so that new, positively reinforcing consequences can be experienced.

Generally speaking, it is in the best interest of the person subjected to punishment for the expression of feelings to limit such expressions.

The behavioral process involved in limiting affective expression is simple avoidance. Just as a rat avoids starting down one runway because it has ended in punishment and instead starts down another, people avoid attending to certain aspects of an evocative situation in favor of attending to others. Technically, one either (1) avoids the conditions that bring about the bodily state (e.g., avoiding having sex), or (2) one does not avoid the precipitating conditions, but instead avoids feeling the bodily state (e.g., "going away" during sex). The client's problems often are the result of this selective avoiding and attending. As a result, the focus of clinical treatment often is on the client's most aversive affective experiences and memories—the very ones that are evoked by situations which the client avoids attending to.

Degree of Contact with Controlling Variables

FAP involves the learning of new behaviors. Behavior, however, cannot be separated from its context. To the FAP therapist, the same behavior in two different contexts has totally different meanings. Therefore, the learning of new behaviors during FAP will serve no purpose unless the context of the session is relevant to daily life. For example, the social skills training approach to assertiveness may or may not be effective. When it does not succeed, it is probably because a new behavior was learned out of the relevant context. That is, the clients were instructed to act assertively in a context different from the one in which their assertiveness was needed. In following the therapist's instructions to be assertive, they are, in fact being compliant. From a FAP standpoint, these clients would have a better chance of learning to be assertive in daily life if they did not want to do the assertion exercise and they refused to do it. Thus, it is important to have the context of daily life operating during the session. The presence of CRB is the best indicator of daily life context. CRB, on the other hand, will be present to the degree that controlling variables are contacted.

What is meant by degree or amount of contact is no more elaborate than the relationship between the salience of a discriminative stimulus (Sd) in a Skinner box and the control exercised by that stimulus. If a dim light is used to signal the availability of food for lever pressing and the light is turned on while the rat is facing away from it, the light will have little or no effect on lever-pressing behavior. Another way of describing the weak relationship between the signal light and the lever press is that the rat is only partially, if at all, in contact with the stimulus. More control over behavior by the Sd would be seen during a subsequent presentation of the light if its intensity were increased and if the rat were oriented toward it. We would then say the rat had more contact with the controlling variables.

As an analogy to the therapy situation in which a client learns to react in a new way, let us say we wanted to change the behavior of the rat in the previous example so that it scratched its head whenever the light came on instead of pressing the lever. The retraining procedure would involve reinforcing scratching only when the light was on. Needless to say, it would be impossible to try to bring scratching under the control of the light and get rid of lever pressing at a time when the rat is not in contact with the light. There would be no training opportunities. This situation is comparable to the difficulty that a client would have in learning new behavior during a session when the relevant controlling stimuli are not present. For example, a client whose problem behaviors only are provoked by intimate situations, will have difficulty in learning new behaviors if the provocative intimate situation does not occur during the session.

Contacting controlling variables can evoke both operant and respondent behavior. For example, the light in the Skinner box concomitantly can serve as a Sd that controls the operant lever pressing and also as a conditioned stimulus that probably elicits salivation and other autonomic changes. Similarly, the client who comes into contact with controlling variables could also show both operant and respondent behavior. For instance, the occurrence of an intimate interaction between the therapist and a client with intimacy problems could produce two simultaneous effects. One could be the showing of feelings involving tears and sadness (respondent), whereas the other could be a CRB involving an attempt to terminate the therapy (operant).

Depending on the degree of contact, the light will have more or less discriminative and eliciting effects and hence more or less effect on the behavior of the rat. Similarly, during FAP a client can have more or less contact with controlling variables. Correspondingly, the client will show more or less of the associated operants or respondents.

In addition to providing new learning opportunities, the limiting of avoidance and increasing contact with controlling variables has the effect of decreasing generalized avoidance and of increasing generalized contact with the world. It is our assumption that avoidance in one area of life has more generalized repercussions that are different for each person. For instance, if one avoids crying, one may also avoid displays of affect in general, and may have difficulty experiencing intense feelings of any kind, including joy and exhilaration.

The case of Jonathan, the second author's client, provides a specific example of how avoidance in a seemingly small area had much greater ramifications. He had been coming to therapy twice a week for over two years and had made tremendous progress—stopped drinking, contacted and worked through the pain of growing up in a dysfunctional family, learned how to describe his feelings, developed a more solid sense of self, and was starting to develop an intimate relationship in which there was a great deal of mutual sharing. He was doing so well that we talked about tapering off his therapy, but one thing nagged at me. When I asked him about his feelings about me, he said he did not have any. He said that he was grateful to me for my help, but that this was strictly a professional relationship and it was not appropriate for him to have feelings for me like he did for other people in his life. I was open to the idea that there were no functional similarities between our relationship and his outside relationships since his other relationships seemed to have improved so much without us having focused very much on ours. But I also told him that I wanted him to explore the possibility that his avoiding having any feelings about me may mean that he was avoiding other things that we were not aware of. We started focusing a lot more on our relationship, and Jonathan agreed to pay more attention to any feelings he had about me. He began reporting that he would notice waking up with warm feelings about me and then immediately he would cut them off. I blocked Jonathan's avoidance by shifting the focus of therapy to his feelings and reactions to me. This led to his having thoughts, such as "I don't deserve to have good feelings, I'll want stuff from you and I'll be disappointed, our relationship will escalate out of control, I'll feel too vulnerable." In the next few months, I encouraged him to keep paying attention to our relationship, to the ways I expressed my caring, and to how he cut off his feelings about me. He gradually came to have more intense feelings about me, and one day he came in and said, "Last night I felt this connectedness in my body and it felt real good. I hadn't felt it for a long, long time [starts getting teary] . . . since I was a kid . . . a feeling of inner purity, being unburdened. I used to be a really nice kid [cries], likable, honest, aware . . . I think I have this general thing, that there are some feelings that aren't okay for me to have, like warm feelings for my Mom, sexual feelings for my shrink, and happy kid-like feelings." Jonathan also reported that he had trouble reaching orgasm during sex, and what he experienced when he was close to orgasm was similar to how he avoided having feelings about me. In short, exploring a limited area of avoidance with Jonathan opened up more realms of experience for him than either of us could have imagined.

The FAP view of emotions can be contrasted with prevalent mentalistic conceptions. Many psychotherapeutic systems and the general public view emotions as something that can be stored, repressed, and discharged. As appealing as these notions are, they leave us with the nagging questions of where they are stored, where they go when they are discharged, and what is left in their place after discharge. Treating emotions as entities leads us to focus on these types of questions and steers us away from their context as part of a person's experience and behavior.

MEMORIES

Clients do two kinds of remembering of early experiences that are useful during psychotherapy. One type occurs spontaneously in the course of conversation. For example, when talking about money owed to the therapist, a client spontaneously remembered that her family was evicted from an apartment building when she was a child because her father had gambled away the rent money. The other type of remembering is directly prompted by the therapist. For example, a client who has some vague recollection about an incest event would be encouraged to think about the event and to remember more about what happened. The behavioral view of these two types of remembering constitutes a somewhat different view from prevailing notions about memories and how they are retrieved. In fact, the radical behaviorist does not believe that there is such a thing as a "memory" that is stored in the mind. We do believe, however, in "remembering" and that this process is important in FAP.

Our view is that remembering is the behavioral process of seeing, hearing, smelling, touching, and tasting of stimuli that are not present. To explain this rather unusual approach to memories, we will discuss only the seeing of stimuli not present since our argument applies equally to the other senses.

Let us start with the notion that seeing is a behavior. When we see a tulip, there is a private activity going on. We cannot describe the activity very well since it is private and we have not learned how to talk about it. It is, however, the private behavior associated with the physiological activity that occurs when we see something. The private activity of seeing, however, is not the physiological activity. Perhaps an analogy to talking will help to clarify this point. Talking is a behavior. Unlike seeing, we can describe talking because it is public and we have learned how to describe this type of public activity. Like seeing, there is a physiological activity associated with talking. As in the case of seeing, however, the talking is not the physiological activity.

Talking provides discriminative stimuli; that is, we can hear the words said and describe jaw movements, and the like. Seeing also provides a complex range of discriminative stimuli. The discriminative stimuli provided by seeing are the object being seen. Thus, the experience we have when we see an object is the result of the discriminative stimuli generated by the behavior of seeing.

Remembering, the behavior of seeing in the absence of an object, can occur in two ways. First, there can be respondently conditioned seeing; that is, the client sees X because X has been associated with other stimuli in the past. For example, consider the word *seven*. For some people, there may have been a brief flash of the numeral 7 in their mind's eye when they saw the printed word. We contend this is an example of respondently conditioned seeing in the absence of the object (the numeral 7) being seen. Similarly, remembering a delicious dinner eaten at a restaurant can be evoked by driving by the restaurant. In the case of Nancy (discussed near the end of this chapter), she spontaneously recalled a previously forgotten separation experience at an aunt's house during childhood. This probably was the result of being in contact with some of the stimuli that were associated with the original trauma. Thus, during the session, there were some separation stimuli (the therapist announced he was leaving for an upcoming vacation) which were associated with the stimuli at the aunt's house, and respondently conditioned seeing (remembering) occurred. This view of remembering is consistent with an extensive literature on state-dependent learning. This literature shows that remembering is facilitated by having stimuli occur in the current situation that are similar to those present when the remembered event first occurred (Catania, 1984). Prior to the recollection, remembering was inhibited because the client avoided contact with the relevant stimuli that both could have elicited the affect and evoked the memory. From this standpoint, then, spontaneous recollections of traumatic events are an automatic effect of contact and serve as an indicator or marker showing the presence of relevant controlling variables. Once contact has occurred, new and more adaptive behavior can be learned. Thus, according to the FAP view, the primary problem that was produced by past trauma is that current stimuli which remind us of the trauma are avoided.

When a client is directly requested to remember an event, this is operant seeing in the absence of the stimulus. Unlike respondently conditioned seeing, which is elicited by a current stimulus that was paired with other stimuli in the past, operant seeing is affected by verbal and other discriminative stimuli, deprivation states, and reinforcement. That is, operant seeing without the stimulus present occurs because of past reinforcement for such visualizing. According to this view, when asked to remember what your bedroom looks like, one simply engages in the same (or similar) private seeing behavior that took place when you were actually were in the bedroom. This seeing is like any other voluntary behavior and its strength will reflect its past reinforcement history. To the degree that the seeing without the stimulus present is similar to the seeing with the stimulus present, the remembering will produce similar discriminative functions.

Thus, if you are trying to recall the exact location of the window or a chair in your bedroom, engaging in the seeing of the bedroom can help in describing exactly where the chair is in much the same manner as seeing the actual bedroom can. The hungry person who imagines food or the sexually deprived one who imagines sexual stimuli are also engaging in operant seeing. In these two instances, deprivation (of food or sex) increases the likelihood of the operant (of seeing food or sex in the absence of a stimulus).

Another implication of operant seeing is that it, like other operants, will not occur if it is punished or otherwise not positively reinforced. Thus, punishment can lead to selective forgetting and amnesia. Selective forgetting and amnesia play a major role in the dissociative disorders such as fugue states and multiple personality disorder (see Chapter 6).

When helping a client to operantly remember an incest event that took place in her bedroom, the client might be first asked to remember the physical features of the bedroom in which the event took place. The client's recalling is shaped and reinforced by the therapist. For example, if remembering the bedroom produces too much aversiveness and is avoided, the client might be asked to recall the hallway leading up to the bedroom.

Remembering early trauma can serve at least two functions. Once a trauma is remembered, the client can then formulate a rule (see Chapter 5) that could help improve functioning in daily life (Zettle, 1980). For example, Zettle described a client who did not enjoy sex with her husband because of forgotten incest. Because the incest was forgotten, the client had formulated an unproductive rule that the sexual problems were due to her husband's ineptness. The rule was unproductive because it led to focusing on the wrong issues and probably led to arguments and frustration. Once the incest was remembered, a new, more productive rule was formulated (e.g., "I am reacting to my husband negatively because of past aversive experiences"), which, in turn, led to a focus on more relevant issues.

A second and more important function of remembering is that it helps to reduce the aversiveness of currently avoided stimuli, and thus helps to increase contact and permit the learning of new, more effective behavior. That is, when the traumatic events are operantly remembered, the aversiveness is reduced by extinction. Then the current stimuli that heretofore were avoided because they elicited respondent seeing will now be contacted. Taking this view of the case example described by Zettle, the operant remembering of the trauma would help because aversiveness is reduced. Then the current sexual relationship would be less likely to be aversive and contact will be improved because the respondent seeing it evokes will be less aversive. This could be expected to directly help improve the sexual relationship.

Correspondingly, operant remembering of past trauma can also increase contact with stimuli within the session, which in turn results in the evocation of CRB. For example, consider a client who presents problems of not trusting others and thus avoids close relationships. The client also avoids trusting and forming a closer relationship with the therapist. Suppose the client then operantly remembers an early abandonment trauma and thereby reduces aversiveness of the remembering. Then the stimuli evoking trust and closeness within the client-therapist relationship, which reminds the client of the abandonment (respondent remembering), would also be reduced in aversiveness. Thus, the CRB2s of trust and closeness are more likely to occur and to be nurtured by the therapist.

Within the FAP framework the avoidance of memories is problematic because it interferes with contact of important stimuli in the client-therapist relationship. Like affect, the spontaneous remembering of traumatic events is a marker indicating contact with clinically significant stimuli within the therapeutic relationship.

CLINICAL IMPLICATIONS

The clinical implications of our theoretical conceptualization of emotions leads to a set of guidelines: (1) offer a behavioral rationale for the importance of affective expression, (2) increase client's private control over feelings, (3) increase therapist affective expression, and (4) enhance client's contact with controlling variables. Some of our methods are similar or identical to techniques from other therapies; the widespread encouragement and facilitation of affective expression as a focus in therapy speak to the usefulness of such expression. Although not necessarily unique, our procedures come from theoretical foundations very different from other therapies. Thus, as the case with many therapies, often *why* we do what we do sets us apart from other systems more than what we actually do. Our guidelines are discussed below.

Offer a Behavioral Rationale for Getting in Touch with Feelings

FAP differs significantly from other views in that the emphasis is not on cathartic release as an end in itself. We believe that avoidance of feelings is accomplished through reduced contact with controlling variables for CRB, which then diminishes the opportunity for acquisition of new behavior. Our explanation to the client of the importance of getting in touch with feelings would not involve appeals of "It's good to get it out, to release those bottled-up feelings," or "If you hold them back they will come out in some other way." Instead, the client would be told that emotion is only an incidental product of dealing with the issues, or of coming into contact with important stimuli. The absence of emotion, however, is a serious problem indicating avoidance which interferes with therapy and also interferes with other areas of the client's life. Thus, emotional expression is crucial not because it is curative by itself, but because it serves as a marker that the client is in touch with important controlling variables, and that new behaviors can now be learned.

In lay terms, to a client who recently went through the ending of a relationship, we might say something like, "It's important to let yourself grieve, because if you avoid thinking, feeling, talking about Jesse, then you end up avoiding a wide range of things, like activities that you did together, or meeting new men, that might bring up any feelings about him. By avoiding all these things, not only is the richness of your life interfered with, but you also don't have the opportunity to figure out what went wrong and to learn new ways of dealing with someone close to you when similar problems come up."

The therapist's response to displays of emotion ideally should be naturally reinforcing. A therapist who has difficulty with his or her own or with other's affective expression is unlikely to offer such encouragement and may punish client affect. Therefore, someone with this type of deficient repertoire would clearly be less able to work well with clients who require increased contact with stimuli evoking emotional responses.

Increase Private Control of Feelings

Frequently, an interaction like the following happens between therapist and client:

T: What are you feeling right now?

C: [*pauses, looks puzzled*] I don't know.

Our interpretation of this comment is based on the stimuli (the environment) that are found in the typical psychotherapy office. The setting is generally benign—the lights are relatively low, the windows are obscured, and the decor is neutral. Usually, client and therapist are seated and inactive except for talking and moving within the confines of the chair. The therapist's facial expressions, gestures, and tone of voice are relatively subdued. Since there is an almost complete absence of public stimuli that might cue clients as to how they are feeling, they must rely almost exclusively on private stimuli. If their past history failed to give them sufficient control by private stimuli, then they will be unable to answer the therapist's question. Thus, the typical therapeutic environment is evocative of the CRB of inadvertent public control of emotions. A goal of treatment for CRB1 associated with inadvertent public control would be aimed at giving private stimuli associated with feelings more control. To accomplish this, first, the therapist would have to be reasonably certain that the relevant bodily states are present and, second, use the principles of discrimination training so that the client's private stimuli (bodily states) would gain control over the description of feelings.

Suppose this type of interaction took place early in the course of therapy, and the client's presenting problem was an inability to express feelings. Further, he has been describing, in monotone, how a co-worker betrayed him. We would encourage him to relive the experience by describing details of the betrayal. Our hope is that his recounting the details would evoke the bodily states of anger. We would also closely observe him to see if there were any signs of anger. Then he might be told "if that happened to me, I would be really angry, and it seems that you might be experiencing some anger right now." After a number of similar therapeutic events in which the client is specifically prompted to tact anger, the specificity of the prompts would be faded. The goal is to have the client's private bodily states gain control of his reports of anger.

From a FAP standpoint, the potency of the therapeutic intervention is strengthened if the emotionally evocative situation actually occurs in the session. For example, suppose a client pleads with the second author to have her call the client's boss to help get a badly needed raise. I refuse, and observe that the client appears disappointed and hurt. At this point, I am reasonably certain that the relevant bodily states of anger are present. Using the principles of discrimination training, initially I would provide salient, public stimuli to prompt the client as to the feeling that should be felt. I might say, "You appear hurt and disappointed, and that's how I would feel if I were in your shoes." Then after numerous instances in which a variety of hurt and disappointment situations have been processed, I gradually would provide less public guidance. Rather than stating specific feelings, I might say, "This situation reminds me of others that you have experienced in the past in which you felt some strong feelings." Still later in the therapy, merely asking the question, "How do you feel?" would be sufficient. An overlap exists between the conditions that lead to a lack of private control of feelings and problems of the self. (This issue and the therapeutic process that leads to increased private stimulus control over the client's responses are discussed in Chapter 6.)

Given how prevalent it is for clients to be unable to answer the therapist when asked how they feel, inadvertent public control of emotions may be more common than generally thought. A lack of clarity over what one is really feeling as an adult, reflects the inevitability of problems that occur when an outside community (e.g., a parent) attempts to impart meaning to an inner experience of the child which they cannot see or know.

Increase Therapist Expression of Feelings

With clients who have difficulty accepting caring from others (the avoidance of expressions of caring feelings by others), and who need help in getting in touch with and expressing their feelings, especially feelings of closeness, we encourage an active expression of feelings by the therapist. For example, the following interaction took place between the second author and Evelyn, her client of four years.

C: [As a kid] I was so ashamed of being poor, of not having anything. My mother humiliated me by being drunk and leaving all the time when she was drunk. No one was healthy enough to be nice. There were never any safe, kind places. I even view you in the same way I used to view people who tried to be nice. It's not real, I'm not really safe, people aren't capable of caring. That's just true. It's too unsafe to trust. At my core, I feel it's not safe.

T: It certainly wasn't safe when you were growing up. About my niceness not being real, last week I asked you to try to feel my caring and you said you felt pain.

C: Yeah, shooting pains, an assault on my barrier. This is the last soldier that's not gonna give up cause a war is still going on. Like those guys you find stalking around in the woods still armed 10 years after the war's over with. To survive all that abuse, this is the last vestige, the belief that the world is still bad. I don't know how to let people love me. That's the secret—I don't know how to do it.

T: You can start by paying attention to the tenderness in my voice, my eyes, my touch, when I talk to you, and by thinking about all the special moments we've had working together all these years.

C: My feeling is, if you really knew me, you wouldn't like me.

T: I know you better than just about anybody, don't I?

C: Yeah.

T: (I move to sit directly in front of her and ask her to look into my eyes while I talk.) Evelyn, when I think about you, there are feelings of warmth and love in my heart. You are very special to me. You've survived so much trauma, and you are a wonderful and talented person. I cherish you and want the very best for you. I consider it a real privilege that you've let yourself be so vulnerable with me, that you've let me get to know who you are, that I've been able to see you change and blossom over the years.

C: [starts crying] It's hard for me to let myself believe you. How come no one else has ever told me this before?

Telling Evelyn how I felt about her served at least four functions. First, this gave her an opportunity to learn, by example, how to express caring feelings. Second, I blocked her avoidance of my expression thereby giving her experience with the accepting of caring feelings from another in a close relationship (CRB2). Third, giving her information about my feelings made me more vulnerable to her. It increased her ability to predict my behavior and thereby to feel safer in the relationship. Finally, telling her my positive feelings toward her should help Evelyn develop more positive self-tacts, such as "I'm a survivor, I'm special, I'm wonderful, I'm talented." These self-tacts could help in the way that cognitive therapy sometimes does (see Chapter 5 for the behavioral account of this phenomenon).

Enhance Client Contact with Controlling Variables

As we have reiterated, bringing clinically relevant behavior (CRBs) into the session is the highest priority for the therapist who is doing

FAP. Sometimes these CRBs do not occur because the client is not sufficiently in contact with controlling variables. In the context of our discussion of emotions, we consider a controlling variable to be anything in the present that reminds someone of emotionally stressful events or trauma that occurred in the past. Examples of controlling variables abound and are, of course, idiosyncratic to the individual. They may include questions or statements made by the therapist, the closeness in the therapy relationship, a picture of a loved one, scenes from a particular movie or book, a specific song, or the twilight hours.

Needless to say, we are most interested in controlling variables that can be brought forth in therapy. Actually, all the preceding examples could have been incorporated into a session. In general, the therapist's task is to enhance the client's contact with controlling variables and to limit the client's avoidance of situations, which occur during the session that evoke affect. When contact occurs, there will be affective expression, which, in turn may evoke more avoidance behaviors.

Thus, the expression of emotion by a client during the session serves as a marker indicating that the client is in contact with the controlling variables that elicit the emotion. Affect serves as a marker indicating contact in the same way that a person who gets close to a hot stove shows actual contact with the stove by (1) crying out in pain, (2) withdrawing from the hot surface, and (3) saying, "(beep) that's hot!" All these expressions of affect are evoked by coming into contact with the hot stove. The bodily state that is felt is the associated experience of pain. If a client is not in contact with relevant controlling variables that would otherwise elicit an emotional response, the marker emotions and associated CRB will not occur.

Note that this analysis of controlling variables and ways of contacting them is an elaboration of Rule 2 (see Chapter 2)—"Evoke CRBs." Three major guidelines that help the therapist to bring the client into contact with controlling variables will now be discussed: (1) Re-present the Aversive Stimulus. (2) Focus on How the Client Is Avoiding Affect. (3) Focus on Client Affect Related to Functional Similarities between Therapy and Daily Life.

Re-present the Aversive Stimulus

Noticing when the client is trying to avoid affect and then re-presenting the relevant aversive stimulus or controlling variable will often block the client's avoidance of affect. Two case studies illustrate this principle.

In the first case, the first author was conducting an initial interview with Amy, a 48-year-old accountant who suffered from unexplained head pain that was present 24 hours a day. Amy was very precise about dates and places, medications, work history, and the like. She was unable, however, to pin down the onset of her pain except to say it started about 8 or 9 years ago and has been present ever since. She appeared to become upset when I persisted in my questions about the date of onset. She was also skillful in changing the topic and did so several times. I took the avoidance as a possible CRB1 and proceeded to push for contact with controlling variables. I asked her to give me an account of all the important events that occurred 8, and then 9 years ago. I wanted to know, for example, what she did for Christmas, what visitors she had during the year, what doctors she saw, if there were any marital problems, etc. As the interview continued and avoidance was blocked time after time, she showed more and more feelings. When I asked her how she felt, she said she felt okay. I took this as evidence that she was not feeling her bodily state very much. I persisted with my questions about significant events during that period of time, and finally she told about the death of her 14-year-old daughter that occurred 8 years ago. She was choked with tears, and her body shook and her arms flailed with anguish. I gently encouraged her to recount in detail the circumstances surrounding her daughter's death. Prior to this catharsis, she completely had avoided any situations that were connected to her daughter's death. She moved to a new home and never went back to the old neighborhood, avoided any discussions which could have led to topics about her daughter, changed her work office, celebrated holidays away from Seattle (her hometown), and never grieved. In many ways her life had become extremely constricted. I saw her a week later and she reported that her head pain had disappeared. My interpretation of Amy's head pain was that it was caused by a chronic bodily state; that is, the pain had a physical origin directly connected to a chronic bodily state that was evoked by the aversiveness of the extensive avoidance.* The events of the session obviated further avoidance and Amy's body returned to a more normal state; the pain disappeared.

The second case example is of Roxie, a client of the second author. Roxie had a history of episodes of severe depressions, suicide attempts, and hallucinations. These intense episodes seemed to be provoked by interpersonal situations in which Roxie was criticized, rebuffed, or oth-

---

*This is an instance in which it can be said that a feeling caused a symptom; that is, the symptom (head pain) was one bodily state which was the direct result of another bodily state (evoked by the aversiveness she was avoiding).

erwise rejected. She would react very emotionally to these events and engage in behaviors such as trying to stab herself with a knife or take an overdose of barbiturates. This was particularly true when the rejection occurred in a relationship that evoked attachment and dependency. After 2 years of therapy marked by many crises, the therapeutic relationship had developed to the point that it approximated the type of relationship that could evoke severe episodes if Roxie experienced a rejection by the therapist. From a FAP standpoint, such an occurrence would provide an invaluable opportunity for the development of more effective ways of dealing with the rejection (CRB2s) and increased self-understanding (CRB3s).

I was reluctantly anticipating just such an opportunity because I was about to tell Roxie that the number and type of evening and week-end phone calls were to be curtailed. When Roxie was told about this limitation, she appeared to be reacting only minimally to the information. She did not cry or act angry but only seemed to be less talkative and changed the topic. It appeared that little contact was made with the situation at hand. It was as if she had not heard or understood what was said. In an effort to bring Roxie into contact with the stimuli that could evoke the emotional response, I brought the conversation back to the topic by stating the limitations again and asking Roxie to repeat what she understood about the phone-call limitation. As Roxie spoke, she became more agitated. With further focusing on the topic and with my stating observations of her avoidance, Roxie began to sob and soon voiced a suicidal thought.

Over the next several months, Roxie gained a greater understanding of the controlling variables (CRB3)—a complex discriminative stimulus involving her attachment to me, the limitation of phone calls, and a history of rejection and abandonment. Also, in the give-and-take of the interaction, she learned a new way of reacting to a rejection. Rather than avoiding and engaging in suicidal behavior, she learned to discuss her dependency and fears of abandonment and to seek reassurance from me. She was gently led to examine which of her behaviors pushed other people away, including me. I tried to give her as much reassurance in words as well as actions about my commitment to her continued growth and improvement. I also persisted in placing limits on the phone calls. The most important lesson for Roxie was that her contacting evocative stimuli in the session resulted in a closer (more reinforcing) relationship. Thus, she was able to experience my caring (reassurance, attention, help in problem solving, etc.) when she also contacted the emotional aspects of having her telephone privileges curtailed. Although it took many months, Roxie was repeatedly brought into contact with the limitation of phone calls and emotional reactions were evoked. This proved to be a turning point in changing how she reacted to rejection and set the stage for the development of other improved interpersonal repertoires.

Focus on How the Client Is Avoiding Affect

In addition to re-presenting the stimulus, another way to enhance contact with controlling variables or to block avoidance is to ask the client to pay direct attention to what she or he is doing so as not to feel. By asking, "What are you doing right now to stop yourself from feeling?" we have found that the major ways clients avoid affect include the following: (1) distractive cognitive activities (e.g., counting backward from 1,000 by sevens, focusing on a blank image, repeating to oneself, "I'm not going to cry"); (2) narrowing one's visual field (e.g., looking intently at something outside the window or a small object in the office like the top button on the therapist's shirt or a speck on the ceiling); and (3) distractive kinesthetic activities (tensing one's muscles, remaining very still, or not breathing). Once we know what they are doing to avoid affect, we ask them to stop doing it or to do something incompatible, like breathing deeply and slowly, or looking into our eyes. Sometimes, simply asking, "Is there something that you're avoiding thinking or talking about right now?" will bring forth an intense topic and its associated affect.

Focus on Client Affect Related to Functional Similarities between Therapy and Daily Life

A functional similarity between therapy and daily life is anything in the therapy situation that would evoke feelings or actions in the client similar to feelings or actions that would be evoked by an outside situation. To illustrate, we turn to the case of Nancy, whose problems centered around forming and maintaining intimate relationships. She had been in FAP with the first author for several months, and an increasingly close relationship was developing. Although progress had occurred, some repertoire deficiencies still remained. One of these, as described by Nancy, concerned a fear that the person she would become close to would disappear, never to return after being temporarily separated from her because of a trip or other such reason. She felt she would be devastated and would not be able to carry on with her life. Nancy saw these feelings as contributing to her past and present reluctance to become intimately involved. This problem also interfered with relationships as they were developing by causing her to feel intense sadness and to withdraw when threatened with separation. She could also relate her fears to having been left by a lover several years before.

Nancy's account of how her fears related to her relationship problems is a description of her problem behavior and possible controlling variables (CRB3). Her account, however, does not constitute an actual occurrence of the problem during the session (CRB1). From a FAP standpoint, the prospects of clinical improvement are enhanced if the fears and associated CRBs provoked by intimacy actually occur within the therapeutic relationship and thereby provide the client an opportunity to learn new ways of responding. Further, a description of her problem behavior and controlling variables that is based on an event occurring during the session would be more beneficial than one based solely on behavior from the client's past.

The marker properties of affect were observed as Nancy's crying when I told her about an upcoming two-week vacation. After reporting an overwhelming sadness, she then attempted to minimize the event, tried to change the topic, and with a smile talked about not needing therapy any longer. I was aware that CRB1 probably was occurring. Therefore, after some words of empathy, I brought the topic back to my upcoming departure. Nancy again became tearful and an intense discussion followed involving our feelings toward each other as well as possible solutions to the immediate problem caused by the vacation, such as having phone contact. In addition, a memory of an early, traumatic experience of being left at an aunt's was recalled by Nancy.

During the session after my return, Nancy reported that she felt much better during my absence than she had anticipated. The interaction was good during that session with both of us feeling closer to each other; this was different from the angry and resentful interactions that usually followed previous reunions with significant others, including me. In the ensuing months, separations from me became less disruptive and, eventually, Nancy reported that she was able to remain stable and not withdraw when anticipating a separation from a person she was becoming involved with. It appeared that new interpersonal repertoires concerning separation within an intimate relationship had been developed.

Nancy's expression of feelings was important in two ways. First, its presence was an indication that the therapeutic situation was functionally similar to her daily life situations involving intimacy and separation. Similar expressions of feelings and withdrawal occurred when the threat of separation occurred in both daily life and in therapy. A therapist who watches for these types of similarities will be more likely to detect CRBs. Second, the disappearance of affect along with the attempt to change the topic was an indication that the client was losing contact with controlling variables. I intervened by bringing up the impending separation again which helped to maintain contact with controlling variables. If contact is maintained, CRB can occur and provide the opportunity for learning improved repertoires.

CASE ILLUSTRATION

Kelly, aged 24, youngest of three children, came into therapy with the first author with the following problems: headaches, depression, chaotic relationships, becoming tearful and similar showings of emotion without any apparent provocation, and feeling awkward, inadequate, incompetent, worthless, and unimportant. Part of her family history involved her father's leaving the family when Kelly was 8 and her seeing him once every 5 years or so. She said she has no feelings and few memories about her father. Her interpersonal history is characterized by social interactions with men from the perspective of whether she is inferior or superior to the person she is talking to. A person who is superior to her can take her or leave her, has little regard for her, does not respect her, and will eventually abandon her. She is attracted to men who are superior to her, but either avoids getting involved with them or has a passionate but stressful relationship which she feels powerless to end but knows she will be left. During the first 4 months of FAP, she was distant and showed little affect. When asked what she thought I felt or thought about her, she replied, "Like a person that you see a lot but you never think about them unless you see them . . . I don't know how to describe it, it's like I am without presence."

Her feeling of being without presence reflects her history. She was not attended to by important men, she was ignored in their presence. It is therefore understandable that she says she feels worthless and unimportant in the therapist's presence. The interaction continued:

T: Well, how do you react to me? (This is a standard FAP question aimed at bringing the tacts under the control of within-session stimuli.)

C: I have this kind of an awe. It's very . . . you're the authority, and it's great that you're seeing me. Yeah. I don't allow myself to be put in the position where I could be hurt. I guess it's like that, but it seems just too cliché that I don't trust anybody, but that's not it as much as somebody seeing me for what I am. I know that at times I really don't come across as that with other people, you know, but I feel inferior. (The client is describing our relationship in a way that sounds similar to how she feels about others in her daily life. She avoids emotional involvement with men who are superior to her because then she can get hurt. Her description is a CRB3. The response is good from a FAP standpoint because it is mainly under the control of within-session stimuli.)

T: Now in our relationship, how would you be hurt by me?

C: Well, there's been a couple times that I've held my breath waiting for you, and you bring something up and I'm not sure what it's leading to. Like you're going to say, "Well I just think that I should stop seeing you, this isn't working." And, it's like I'm waiting for the axe to fall at all times.

(Kelly becomes tearful at this point. In talking about our relationship, she is contacting evocative stimuli associated with being abandoned. She is tacting her feelings that are evoked in the session. Because of her early abandonment, she avoids getting into this kind of situation during her daily life. This avoidance contributes to her relationship problems. Her affect suggests that the client-therapist relationship provides an opportunity to overcome her avoidance and fear by repeated contacting of the evocative stimulus, experiencing a better outcome than in her past, and thereby improve her relationships in daily life.)

(A few minutes later)

T: You were kind of tearful before, right?

C: Yeah. I get like that a lot. I get upset and I just get choked up.

T: There must be something that came up in our conversation, from what we were talking about that got to you. (I am suggesting that external variables, something about our interaction, were responsible for her emotional response.)

C: Yeah.

T: And you don't know what it is?

C: No I don't.

T: So there is kind of like an emotional trigger in there and you're not sure what starts the trigger going.

C: When I saw my father for the first time since I was 15, which was when I was 19 or 20, I must have cried for two days. I mean literally buckets, I just couldn't stop crying. I was even laughing through it and I thought . . . well, anyway. (This is remembering that was evoked by events occurring in the session which also evoked responses similar to those in the recalled situation.)

(Later in the same session)

T: There's some kind of emotional trigger in here that, no doubt, was caused by your relationship with your father, that came up between us just before. You're walking around with a reaction in you that you don't understand and can't anticipate occurring. (I am offering an interpretation—Rule 5.)

Over the course of the next 2 years, CRB related to her fears and memories about her father continued to occur as Kelly formed a closer relationship with me. During this time, I openly expressed my feelings (including my high regard for her) and expressed them in the same manner that she was encouraged to do.

As discussed previously, the therapist's expression of feelings has several positive effects. In this case, I became more predictable to Kelly and she knew better what to expect, a contrast from most of her previous relationships which were experienced as dangerously unpredictable. Her being able to predict my behavior better, in turn, reduced her avoidance and facilitated her expression of feelings. Correspondingly, she experienced this as an increased trust in me. Furthermore, my openness and positive statements spontaneously increased as she became more emotionally expressive, thus providing natural reinforcement for her improvements. Her increased emotional expression along with my acceptance of it encouraged an improved self (see Chapter 6). There were also many discussions about the features of our relationship and each of our repertoires that made it so reinforcing (Rule 5, CRB3). These verbal descriptions helped Kelly in knowing specifically what to expect in a good relationship. The positive experience of our relationship allowed her to look for similar positive relationships in her daily life.

Toward the end of Kelly's therapy, she was relaxed and confident during the sessions. She related to me as an equal and was not in awe of me. She valued our relationship and saw herself as being important to me. Her relationships with men also reflected this improvement.

5

Cognitions and Beliefs

Harriet was asked by the first author to change her regular appointment time from 5:00 PM Mondays to 3:00 PM Tuesdays. Although she consented, Harriet revealed several weeks later that the change had caused a great deal of hardship. In order to accommodate the change, she had had to rearrange her work and school schedules, and her presenting problems of anxiety and depression were exacerbated. When asked why she did not refuse my request or explain how the change would be difficult, Harriet gave the following interpretation. Although it had occurred to her to object, she thought, "My willingness to give in to you shows how much I care about you and, besides, I didn't want you to get angry at me. I can't stand to have people I care about get angry at me."

Like Harriet, clients often describe and/or act in ways that suggest a causal relationship between their thoughts and feelings and their behavior. The therapist's view on the nature of the causal relationship between thoughts (or cognitions) and behavior (or actions and feelings) is important because it enters into what is said and done in the course of therapy. Nowhere is this more apparent than in the widely used procedures of cognitive therapy. Since many therapists are familiar with the tenets of cognitive therapy, we will use it as the basis of comparison, highlighting the similarities and differences to functional analytic psychotherapy (FAP). In general, we believe cognitive therapy is a useful treatment that can be improved with the addition of FAP theory and practice.

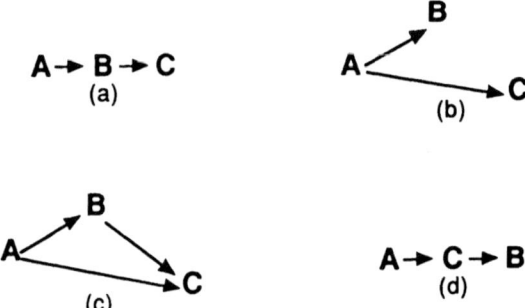

Figure 2. Paradigms showing relationships between *A* (antecedent event), *B* (belief or think-ing), and *C* (consequent behavior or feeling): (a) thinking influences behavior; (b) thinking has no influence on behavior; (c) thinking partially influences behavior; and (d) behavior influences thinking.

COGNITIVE THERAPY

Considerable diversity exists in the underlying theory and practice of cognitive therapy, and the precise manner in which the thought-be-havior relationship is stated depends on the particular orientation and how thoughts are conceptualized. For example, Albert Ellis (1962, 1970), a pioneer in cognitive therapy, introduced the idea that a client's thoughts and feelings could be represented by Figure 2a, in which *A* represents external environmental events, *B* represents cognition, and *C* is the re-sulting action and/or emotion. For Ellis, clinical treatment involved giving clients the *ABC* explanation of their problems and then directing attempts to change *B* so that it was no longer dysfunctional.

Since there are problems with this *ABC* paradigm, accordingly, it has been revised (Beck, Rush, Shaw, & Emery, 1979; Guidano & Liotti 1983; Hollon & Kriss, 1984; Turk & Salovey, 1985). It is our opinion, however, that the revised cognitive therapy formulation has thrown out the baby with the bathwater; that is, it loses some of the clinically useful features of the *ABC* formulation and has not adequately addressed the problems. Before looking at the revised view of cognitive therapy, let us briefly examine some of the problems with cognitive therapy and the *ABC* formulation.

Problems with Cognitive Therapy and the *ABC* Paradigm

First, the *ABC* paradigm excludes alternative ways in which cogni-tion and behavior could be related. For example, Russell and Brandsma

(1974) suggested that client problems could start out fitting the $A \rightarrow B \rightarrow C$ paradigm. Then, after numerous repetitions of the ABC sequence during the client's life, classical conditioning would obviate the occurrence of B. In other words, A becomes a second-order conditioned stimulus that directly elicits C. Another possibility, suggested by Klein (1974), is that the depressed patient's negative self-concept, helplessness, and self-blame are best viewed as an effect rather than a cause of the condition. In other words, the client first feels depressed and then has the negative cognitions.

Clinical experience also suggests alternative paradigms. When clients make such comments as "I intellectually accept that I don't need to be loved by everyone but I still feel devastated when I'm rejected," they report the presence of a B that is inconsistent with the C. On the other hand, some clients claim that they experience no conscious B that precedes their problematic C, thus indicating that there is no B, or that the B is unconscious.

A second problem with the ABC paradigm is that its use in therapy can lead to some questionable clinical procedures. For example, if the cognitive therapist truly believes the ABC hypothesis, the client's rejection of it is challenged. The challenge takes the form of directly questioning the client's logic or sincerity, or by proposing that there are additional, unconscious cognitions to be discovered. Challenges can also be indirect. Rather than confront the client's rejection of the ABC model in the session, the therapist gives instead additional homework or assumption-testing assignments. This nonacceptance of alternative paradigms is found in the cognitive therapy of Aaron Beck (1976), even though he rejects the theory implied by the ABC model. For example, Beck suggested that clients who say that they intellectually "know" they are not worthless, but who do not accept this on an emotional level, need more cognitive therapy because the dysfunctional feelings can only occur when they do not "truly believe" the rational thought (Beck et al., 1979, p. 302). The prescription of "more cognitive therapy" is an indirect way of challenging the client's rejection of the ABC model.

Given the complexity of human behavior, the exclusion of coexistent, noncognitive mediated explanations as demanded by the ABC model seems unreasonable.

From a FAP standpoint, an antitherapeutic effect of the ABC model could occur when a client who does not accept the ABC theory is challenged by the therapist. If this client were seeking help with becoming more assertive or with having more confidence in his or her own opinions, then objecting to the therapist's ABC theory could be a desirable behavior. Ideally, this within-session improvement should be reinforced by the therapist's acceptance and not punished by the challenges.

A third problem with the *ABC* paradigm concerns the evidence used to support the notion that dysfunctional feelings and actions are caused by deviant, irrational, or pathological *B*s. One type of supportive evidence can be gathered by comparing the thoughts and attributions of clients to "normal" subjects (for a recent review, see Beidel & Turner, 1986).

Not surprisingly, clients tend to have more dysfunctional thoughts than do normals. Such research is problematic because it only demonstrates that people with clinical problems also have irrational thoughts and does not demonstrate that the thoughts actually cause the problems. In addition to supporting the causal status of cognitions, such data equally support the notion that cognitions are caused by the dysfunctional feelings and actions, or that both the cognitions and the actions/feelings are caused by some third variable. Some data even indicate that depressed persons may assess reality more accurately than normals (Krantz, 1985). These data are inconsistent with an *ABC* explanation for depression in which the *B* is defined as a distorted or deviant view of reality. A recent review of the experimental literature on the relation between internal states and actions also supports the notion that *B* (the internal state) and *C* (the action) are sometimes not congruent (Quattrone, 1985).

A fourth problem concerns the theory-practice connection. It is unclear how the cognitive hypothesis is related to many of the specific treatment procedures. Why and how, for example, does logical argument or evidence change a cognitive structure? How does cognitive theory support Beck's advocation of a Socratic approach in which clients must discover for themselves their underlying assumptions? How is it relevant to Ellis's direct instruction to clients to adapt new beliefs? What are the theoretical principles involved in accounting for cognitive change as a result of clients' performing experiments in their daily lives to check out hypotheses? How does the client's talking about cognitions and their relation to symptoms (metacognition) help to change structures? How is it possible to have cognitive therapies that are not metacognitive (Hollon & Kriss, 1984)? That cognitive therapy is effective is not an issue. What is problematic is the adequacy of the theory to account for treatment outcome. As expressed by Silverman, Silverman, and Eardley (1984, p. 1112), the clinical effects that occur as a result of cognitive therapy are "awaiting for a convincing rationale."

Revised Formulation of Cognitive Therapy

As a step toward improving the *ABC* model, cognitive therapists have turned to basic cognitive theory and have revised or more precisely specified what is meant by *B* (cognition) and how it is related to clinical problems. For example, Hollon and Kriss (1984) delineated the different uses of the term *cognition* and distinguished between *cognitive products* and *cognitive structures* (and associated *cognitive processes*).* Cognitive products are directly accessible, conscious, private behaviors, such as thoughts, self-statements, and automatic thoughts. Cognitive structures, for instance, "schemas," are the underlying organizational entities that play an active role in processing information. Structures, however, operate at an unconscious level since their content cannot be known directly and must be inferred from the products.

As pointed out by Hollon and Kriss, this distinction is similar to the difference between the linguist's surface and deep structures. Surface structures refer to what is said (overt verbalizations) or thought (covert self-statements), whereas deep structures refer to what is meant. From the Hollon and Kriss perspective, the causal factor is the cognitive structure, whereas the thinking or the cognitive products (irrational thoughts, self-statements, automatic thoughts) constitute "signs or hints of the nature of one's knowledge structures."

Therefore, Hollon and Kriss suggested that any clinical interventions that change cognitive products are merely symptomatic treatments. In a similar vein, Safran, Vallis, Segal, and Shaw (1986) warned that changing products has limited clinical effects, and efforts should be directed at "core" processes. Correspondingly, Beck (1984) warned that relapse can be expected unless underlying cognitive structures are changed and has stated that the notion that cognitive phenomena cause depression is "far-fetched." Presumably, the "cognitive phenomena" whose causality Beck rejected are cognitive products, whereas core structures or schema are still viewed as causal.

Although in the theoretical realm the causality of cognitive products has been replaced by structures, a corresponding shift has not occurred in the trenches where cognitive therapy is actually practiced. The same cognitive therapists who reject the causative role of cognitive products are the ones who provide cognitive therapy treatment manuals and clini-

---

*Structures and processes are not differentiated in this book because the distinctions between them do not affect our analysis.

cal examples that focus on changing cognitive products. For example, Beck, Emery, and Greenberg (1986) stated that the therapist "must be able to communicate clearly that anxiety is maintained by mistaken or dysfunctional appraisal of a situation" and "gives this explanation . . . in the first session and reiterates it throughout therapy" (p. 168). Guidano and Liotti (1983, pp. 138-142) stated that first important step in therapy occurs "when patients understand that their suffering is mediated by their own opinions."

If clinical practice followed the shift in cognitive theory, the obvious focus would be on changing the "underlying" structures. From a behavioral point of view, the theory-practice schism in cognitive therapy makes sense. Since the only contact the therapist has with the client is with his or her behavior, and since cognitive products are defined in terms of behavior, the clinical intervention can be specified as a *behavior change process*. Cognitive structures, however, are defined as nonbehavioral entities that cannot be contacted by the therapist. Since clinical interventions are always limited to the behavioral realm—the client's thinking, feeling, talking, theorizing, free-associating, and the like—it is impossible to devise treatments that focus on structures which do not involve these client behaviors. Thus, it is difficult to come up with interventions aimed at structures that are different from those aimed at products.

For example, Beck *et al.* (1979) stated that "the cognitive and behavioral interventions [used] to modify thoughts . . . are the same as those . . . used to change hidden assumptions" (p. 252). The only procedures that differentiate the clinical treatment of products from structures is that the latter must first be inferred (e.g., the client must abstract or deduce the existence of the structure). Once identified, however, the same therapeutic methods used to change products are applied. Directed by theory to change a nonbehavioral entity (the underlying structure), while restricted to working with the behavior (products) of the client, the practicing cognitive therapist is in an untenable position. These theoretically posited difficulties in changing schemas and the tenuous link between theory and how change occurs has been termed a dilemma by Hollon and Kriss (1984, pp. 46-48). Although they and such other cognitive psychologists as Guidano and Liotti (1983) are working on finding ways out of this dilemma, the jury is out as to whether satisfactory resolutions have or can be developed. It is not surprising, therefore, that the actual nuts-and-bolts practice of therapy seems, of necessity, to focus on products.

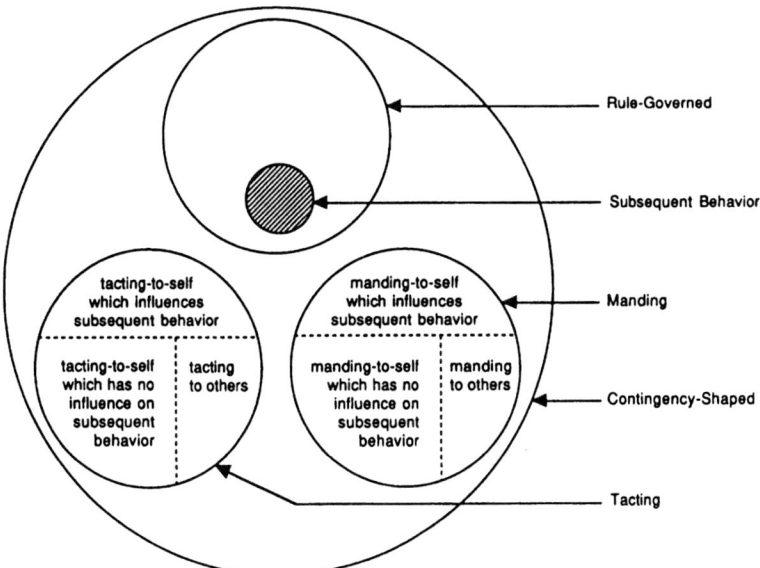

Figure 3. Types of verbal behavior that may or may not influence subsequent behavior. Tacting-to-self and manding-to-self, which influence subsequent behavior, lead to a subset of rule-governed behavior (shaded area).

THE FAP REVISION OF $A \rightarrow B \rightarrow C$

As an alternative, we have proposed a formulation of the thought-behavior relationship that retains the clinical usefulness but avoids the problems of the original ABC hypothesis. According to our model, cognitions can play either a major, minor, or no role in the client's problems. Correspondingly, cognitive therapy methods will be of varying effectiveness with different clients depending on the role that cognition has in the clinical problem. Our behavioral conception of cognition involves several different types of client behavior including contingency-shaped behavior, rule-governed behavior, and two types of verbal behavior, "tacts" and "mands." As shown in Figure 3, they overlap one another in varying degrees. Of particular importance to this analysis are tacting-to-self and manding-to-self behaviors. Before explaining our model, we will elaborate on the concepts of tact-, mand-, and contingency-shaped behavior that were previously discussed in Chapter 3.

Contingency-Shaped Behavior

As pointed out previously, contingency-shaped behaviors are those behaviors which have been directly strengthened by reinforcement. Many behaviors, however, have not been directly reinforced and instead are more a function of the prior stimulus. For example, instructions are a prior stimulus that can evoke complex behaviors which have never before been directly reinforced. Similarly, an instructor demonstrating what to do can evoke behavior not previously reinforced. In these cases, the contingencies have shaped the more global behavior (e.g., imitating the instructor or following instructions), but have not yet had a chance to exert much influence on the specific behavior being imitated or the instructed behavior. Thus, all behavior is ultimately contingency-shaped.

Even though a conscious experience of pleasure may often accompany contingencies involving positive reinforcement, it is not a necessary part of the shaping and strengthening process and should not be confused with it. Almost all of our behavior (e.g., talking, walking, running, etc.) is there because of the strengthening effects of reinforcement, and these behaviors were strengthened mostly without our awareness of the process. Conscious experiences (to be discussed later) do play an important albeit different role from that of behavior which is directly shaped by contingencies. However, the fact that conscious experience is more directly felt than the unconscious effects of reinforcement can easily lead to the latter's being overlooked.

One way to look at Harriet's behavior (described in the example above) is that her acquiescence was purely contingency-shaped and was not influenced by her preceding thoughts. From this standpoint, her acquiescence would have been shaped directly by experiences with people's anger when she inconvenienced them. These experiences could have occurred in childhood and/or at preverbal infancy. They would have included the punishment of being told "no" or other types of non-verbal refusal, the reinforcement of acquiescence, and the lack of accommodation from others contingent on making her wishes known. This resulted in certain responses (acquiescence) being stronger than others (assertiveness). Thus, acquiescing is seen as the direct result of contingencies and would be expected to occur again under the right conditions, such as those that occurred in the therapy session. Even though such contingencies can have these particular effects, this does not mean that the client is aware or conscious of the process. Thus, it is quite possible that Harriet is unaware or unconscious of the causes of her behavior. In terms of the *ABC* paradigm, contingency-shaped behavior would correspond to $A \rightarrow C$. The fact that other people would respond differently to the same *A* reflects the difference in their past experiences when in *A* situations.

Tacts and Mands: Two Types of Verbal Behavior

The contingency-shaped explanation, however, does not account for *B*, the thinking that Harriet described. In order to explain how Harriet came to have her thoughts, we return to tacts and mands, two types of verbal behavior.

To review, tacts include the labeling and describing of events and objects. Examples of tacts are "That is water," "I screamed at him," and "I can't stand this."

Mands, on the other hand, include commands, threats, and requests. The defining characteristic of a mand is that it is strengthened by a very narrow range of contingencies. For example, the mand, "I would like some water" will be strengthened only if it results in the listener's providing water or some other thirst quencher.

According to the behavior analytic position, tacts and mands are learned in the same way that any other behaviors are learned. Thus, when and how we tact or mand varies from person to person depending on their particular experiences. As an example of how tacting is acquired, consider a child who learns to say "truck" when one goes by because that is how the parent described it. The child is reinforced directly ("that's right, that's a truck") and indirectly as "truck" enters into other contexts (the child says, "I want a truck" or "Give me that truck"). In the same way that one learns to describe inanimate objects or such past events as "it rained last Tuesday," one also learns to describe others' and one's own present behavior and past experiences. A man who approaches the dentist's chair and says, "This is going to hurt and I am afraid" is probably tacting (1) past experiences of being hurt by dentists, (2) his feelings of fear (see Chapter 4 for a behavioral view of feelings and what is "felt"), and (3) a prediction of how he is going to react when in the chair.

Up to this point, the tacting and manding we have discussed have been said out loud to another person. Whether said out loud or to oneself, however, we all know that tacting and manding also occur when the only person hearing the description or demand is the speaker. From our standpoint, tacting and manding to oneself is functionally the same as tacting and manding out loud when no other person is present. These two cases differ mainly in the intensity of the response. We are particularly interested in tacting and manding to oneself because this is also known as *thinking*. Thus, our definition of thinking is tacting and mand-ing to oneself.

The question we will now address is why thinking (and the similar tacting and manding out loud without a listening audience) occurs; that is, we have explained why a person would tact and mand when others can hear, as in "This is terrible," "I'm anxious," "Be patient," "Keep your mouth shut," "Get out of bed," and "Do it now." It is less clear why these would be thought or said aloud when no one is around.

We are particularly interested in tacting-to-self and manding-to-self because they often encompass what is meant by *B* in cognitive therapy. For example, the words *must* and *should* are viewed as a cause of neurosis by rational emotive therapists, and their clinical interventions are aimed at eliminating such words from their client's thinking (Ellis, 1970). Typi-cally, these words (must and should) are also found in manding-to-self statements, such as "I must never make mistakes" and "I should be happy." Similarly, "I am unlovable" would be viewed by cognitive thera-pists as an irrational thought or dysfunctional hypothesis that causes client problems. The thought "I am unlovable" is a tact made to oneself. Therefore, a behavioral explanation of why tacting-to-self and manding-to-self occur and how they affect client problems is important in our account of cognition and cognitive therapy.

Generalized Tacts and Mands That Have No Influence on Subsequent Behavior

We believe that the *ABC* model encompasses several types of *B-C* relationships. The first case we will consider is an absence of relationship between *B* and *C*, which occurs when tacting-to-self or manding-to-self is simply due to stimulus generalization and not because it affects sub-sequent behavior. Thus, we are so used to tacting or manding to others that some persistence would be expected when we are alone (e.g., a child saying out loud "truck" even when a parent is not around). Generali-zation from public reactions to the private realm is particularly expected to occur if its public form is strong. For example, the considerable strength of manding-to-others is illustrated by its frequent generalization to inanimate objects, such as shouting "start!" to a stalled car or scream-ing warnings of a blitz to a football team on television. Obviously, these tacts and mands have no effects on the objects. Another example of manding without an audience that occurs because of generalization of a high-strength behavior is observed in the Kaingang Indians, who shout at thunderstorms to make them go away (Skinner, 1957). Skinner ac-counted for this behavior in terms of its resemblance to that of shouting at men to make them go away as well as the adventitious reinforcement of the storms' eventually moving on.

Let us return to the case of Harriet and describe how she could have thoughts (a behavior) that appear to be linked causally to another subsequent behavior when in reality they are not linked. In this illustration, we posit that her thinking is tacting-to-self due to generalization and her acquiescing has been purely contingency-shaped. In order for Harriet to tact-to-self due to generalization, she would have had a history in which she learned to describe her own behavior and experiences to others, such as telling her mother, "When I said no, daddy got angry" (a tact). Then, because of stimulus generalization she engages in similar behaviors when others are not around (e.g., tacting recent experiences). We are surmising that Dad did not reinforce Harriet for saying no to him and did reinforce her compliance with his requests. As these contingencies (Dad's reactions) were directly shaping her acquiescence behavior pattern and evoking associated feelings, she also described to herself the contingencies (e.g., "Daddy just pushed me away when I asked him for attention") and her own operant and respondent behaviors ("I ran to my room and started to cry"). Thus, at the same time that the acquiescence and lack of assertiveness were being shaped, she also described to herself the events as they were unfolding. She thought and acquiesced; the thinking and acquiescing were independent of each other. Now, in similar situations Harriet will similarly engage in both behaviors; that is, she will think and acquiesce. In terms of the ABC paradigm, these actions are represented by Figure 2b. It just so happens that the B precedes the C in time, but B has no effect on C.

The combinations of the two separate behaviors, contingency-shaped acquiescence and generalization-induced tacting-to-self or manding-to-self, offer an account of how a person can have thoughts (thinking behavior) and behavior (a subsequent behavior) that are not causally linked although they may appear to be. If this set of circumstances actually occurs for some clients, it would be a mistake to take their thoughts as causal, to fit them into an ABC paradigm, and (compounding the error) to ignore the role that contingencies played in forming the behavior.

Generalized Tacts and Mands That Influence Subsequent Behavior

Up to this point, we have looked at thinking as behavior that does not enter into the causal chain of events leading to C. Now we will examine circumstances in which tacting-to-self and manding-to-self can have considerable effect on subsequent behavior. Before we do so, however, it is important to clarify a semantic problem concerning the word *cause*. Cognitive psychologists and radical behaviorists mean different things when they refer to cause. To the cognitive psychologist, the effect of one's thoughts on behavior represents a type of causal relationship (whether it be partial, contributory, or otherwise). The term *cause* simply means that thoughts are considered to bring about a change in behavior. To the radical behaviorist, the term *cause* is limited to the effects of contingencies. The same effects that are called *causal* by cognitivists, that is, the effects of thoughts on the behavior that follows, are seen to exist but are described differently by radical behaviorists.

For example, Skinner (1957) spoke of private events being "helpful" or "speed[ing] acquisition" (p. 445) and having "practical effects" (p. 440). In his discussion on formulating a rule to guide one's own behavior, Skinner (1969) also talked about a person who formulated tacts-to-self because he himself could then react more "effectively" (p. 159). Hayes (1987), when speaking of the thought-behavior relationship, referred to the kinds of contingencies that would lead one behavior to occur and to, in turn, "influence" another behavior (p. 331). Thus, it appears that both cognitive and radical behaviorists observe a similar phenomenon but use different terms to describe it. Perhaps some of the conflict between the two positions is due to this difference.

Tacting-to-self can be useful to the individual who does it when it helps to clarify or identify a situation that might otherwise be confusing. For example, the first author was seeing a female client who unpredictably became hostile at times during the sessions. Several different conditions lead to her hostility, including (1) if her interactions with her husband had gone well that week and she felt I was too confrontive and expecting too much from her during the session; (2) if she had a bad week with her husband and viewed me as being too distant and not involved; and (3) if she felt I was being too obsequious. Making these interpretations to the client (Rule 5) were not useful at this point in her therapy and only evoked more hostility. Interpretations were useful, however, when made to myself. The tacting-to-self helped me to figure out how to respond to the hostility in a therapeutic way. Most human interactions are quite complex, and how one tacts (labels, categorizes, or classifies) the situation can help in determining an effective reaction.

Similarly, manding-to-self might increase a person's effectiveness at the task at hand. Such a case is illustrated in Skinner's observations of a little girl who talked out loud to herself while practicing the piano —"No, wait," "Just a minute," and "Is that right?" (1957, p. 444). Such mands-to-self may have helped strengthen the subsequent behaviors of stopping and listening. Originally, the child said these mands due to generalization from hearing them from others and saying to others the very same statements. Eventually, with enough experience, the contingencies of improved piano-playing (e.g., the useful purpose) will influence whether or not the child continues to make and follow these mands to herself (whether out loud or in thought). Another comment or tact-to-self by the child was, "That's in the key of G". Such a description could have helped reduce errors in much the same way that the same statement made by her teacher would have.

Although the present section is about thoughts that affect subsequent behavior, Skinner made additional observations of the little girl that illustrate the case previously discussed in which thoughts have no effect. The little girl also said, "My finger it hurts so much," and told the clock "Don't do that! You're going too fast!" Skinner speculated that these statements had no effect on her subsequent piano-playing behavior. Thus, while observing the same child doing the same task, Skinner suggested that some of her tacting-to-self and manding-to-self did affect subsequent behavior and some did not. This corresponds to the FAP view of client thoughts. Further, the tacting-to-self and manding-to-self, which does lead to useful strengthening of behavior, contributes to maintaining generalization so that it will also occur even when it has no effects on subsequent behavior.

The case in which tacting-to-self and manding-to-self does lead to useful strengthening of subsequent behavior will now be applied to Harriet's case. Suppose that Harriet had learned to describe certain requests made by others (no matter how innocuous) as a test of her love for them. She could have learned this as a child from her narcissistic mother who often needed affirmations of love, and who would ask questions with a hidden agenda. For example, when her mother asked, "Did you like the pie I made for you," the question had little to do with the taste of the pie. Instead she really meant, "Do you love me and appreciate what I do?" "If you don't, I will get depressed and withdraw."

On account of a child's difficulty in discriminating a "real" question from a test one, Harriet might have experienced unpredictable punishment and reward. Furthermore, suppose that she discussed this problem with friends or a therapist and obtained an awareness or insight into the conditions that differentiated an ordinary question from a "test" question. Thereafter, when confronted with a question, Harriet would privately review (tact) the conditions in order to decide (discriminate) whether or not it was a test. Then, to herself, she might say, "This is a test of love. If I act in a way that is rejecting, she will get angry; if I go along with the program, she will be happy." In terms of the *ABC* paradigm, this continuation is represented in Figure 2a.

Of course, this description of Harriet's thinking corresponds more closely to the cognitive therapy paradigm in which *B* is a cognitive product, such as conscious experiences of thoughts or self-statements. Such a model assumes that there is little or no independently shaped or conditioned *C*.

Our position, however, is that even though Harriet's behavior was influenced by her thinking and thus corresponds to the $A \rightarrow B \rightarrow C$ paradigm, she would, in time, experience the success or failure of her decision process. Then her acquiescence would be influenced more by the unconscious effects of the contingencies and less by the conscious "decision process." This process in which contingency-shaped behaviors and tacting-to-self and manding-to-self start out as independent, but then come to interact with each other, represents another possible arrangement of the thought-behavior relationship. Thus, in time, a reaction that is first brought about by tacting-to-self or manding-to-self would become contingency-shaped.

A slightly different interpretation of Harriet's thinking is to view *C* as contingency-shaped and, in addition, to posit a *B* that also strengthens *C*. In other words, Harriet could have had the unconscious effects of reinforcement that made her acquiescence more likely and, at the same time, engaged in a conscious tacting-to-herself that would strengthen her acquiescing. In this case, the *C* would be stronger than the *C* that is just contingency-shaped or one that only evoked by *B*. This paradigm is represented in Figure 2c.

The behavioral formulations of thought-behavior relations discussed so far do not exhaust all possibilities. It is possible to have the case like that represented in Figure 2d, in which emotional reactions and/or behavior are directly evoked and then, in James-Lange fashion, clients figure out what they must have been thinking. It is also possible for the occurrence of an independent *B* to have an effect on subsequent behavior because of a consistency effect, which occurs in people who have learned that "one should practice what one preaches" or "not say one thing and do another." In the case of consistency, thoughts influence subsequent behavior because these individuals have been reinforced for doing what they said they would do, and punished when their actions were not consistent with their verbal behavior.

It is also important to mention some of the special problems engendered by the fact that *B*s cannot be observed directly and must either be inferred or based on self-descriptions. Thus, it is possible that a self-description of a *B*, like the one given by Harriet, may be a mere fabrication or one that is required by social convention. Even in those cases where the client is giving his or her best description of B, such introspection is known to be unreliable and subject to many current influences.

Although a complete account of thought-behavior relationships would include these as well as other paradigms and influencing factors, the FAP account and some of its major theoretical implications are conveyed by the paradigms delineated above.

Rule-Governed Behavior

We will now discuss the relationship between rules, rule-governed behavior, and tacting-to-self and manding-to-self. We are introducing this topic because the literature on rules and rule-governed behavior (Skinner, 1969; Zettle & Hayes, 1982) is relevant to our concept of the thought-behavior relationship and further clarifies the issues.

When a tact or mand specifies a contingency and the behavior required, it is referred to as a *rule*. For example, the statement "If you were more friendly, you would have friends" is a tact that is a rule because it is a description specifying a behavior (being friendly) and a contingency (having friends). "You must do your homework assignments or leave therapy" is a mand that is a rule because it is a demand specifying a behavior (doing homework) and a contingency (terminating therapy). Thus, laws, logical principles, instruction manuals, injunctions, maxims, and threats are tacts and mands which are also rules. The example of Harriet's tacting-to-self is an instance of a rule because it specifies the required behavior (acquiescence) and the contingencies (avoid trouble). The behavior that occurs as a result of the rule being issued is referred to as *rule-governed behavior*. For example, a mother issues a rule when she tacts to her son "If you don't get out of bed now, you will be late for school." The son's getting out of bed would then be rule-governed behavior. After a rule is issued, rule-governed behavior may or may not occur. Thus, you might tell yourself that you must finish the paper you are writing tonight or you will feel terrible. Even though this mand-to-self is a rule, it may or may not result in rule-governed behavior (i.e., you may or may not finish the paper).

Rule-governed behavior would never occur unless the individual had been reinforced, in general, for the act of following rules. This reinforcement occurs from childhood on as we are given innumerable rules in the form of "If you do (or don't do) such and such, then this and that will happen to you." Obviously, there much variability in how accurate the rule is. For some children, their parents give accurate rules, and when the children follow the rule, the specified consequence occurs. For other children, the rules are not accurate and the child learns to ignore them. For example, graduate students probably have early histories in which they were reinforced for following rules, particularly those that are found in the classroom. Surely, they are examples of persons who have been reinforced for following the instructions and teachings of professors. The specific behavior evoked by the rule, however, may never have been reinforced. Thus, a student may do a complex set of actions, such as designing, running, and analyzing dissertation research, that has not been contingency-shaped but is rule-governed. Eventually, however, the contingencies will prevail as is the case with all rule-governed behavior. If the contingencies of doing the dissertation are positive (such as finding interesting and worthwhile results which set the stage for further research), the student may become a prolific researcher. If the contingencies are punitive (such as finding equivocal, meaningless results requiring endless statistical analysis), he or she may never again do research after the dissertation.

As discussed for tacts and mands, rules are extracted from one's own or others' direct experience of the contingencies of reinforcement or from the study of the systems that arrange them. The development of rule-extracting and rule-governed behavior becomes a large part of one's behavior because it helps to shorten the tedious process of shaping. The tacting-to-self that Harriet developed is an example.

It is difficult to tell if a person is acting on the basis of rules ($A \rightarrow B \rightarrow C$) or contingencies ($A \rightarrow C$) just by looking at the action itself. For example, a poker player who figures out the odds to himself before making a play ($A \rightarrow B \rightarrow C$) might make the same actions as another player who has been shaped by the contingencies ($A \rightarrow C$), but their controlling variables are fundamentally different. Thus, one player is thinking about what to do before he does it and the other is probably relying on feeling or intuition, which is the experiential aspect of previous reinforcement history. Correspondingly, the effectiveness of any intervention aimed at changing behavior would depend on whether the behavior to be changed is an $A \rightarrow C$ or an $A \rightarrow B \rightarrow C$ type. If, for example, you wished to change either card player's behavior, the one who figures the odds might be more influenced by new methods of figuring odds taught at a gambling school than would the contingency-shaped player.

The distinction between rule-governed and contingency-shaped behavior is used by Skinner (1974) in his reconceptualization of many common polarizations. Some of these are: deliberation versus impulse, contrived versus natural, intellect versus emotion, logic versus intuition, conscious versus unconscious, surface versus depth, and truth versus belief. In a similar way, Skinner's distinction between contingency-shaped behavior and rule-governed behavior bears a striking resemblance to cognitive therapy's distinction between cognitive products and structures.

Cognitive Structures and Contingency-Shaped Behavior

As pointed out earlier, some forms of cognitive therapy underscore the importance of changing structures (as opposed to products), yet lack theoretically based means for doing so. Since behavior analysis is primarily a theory of behavior change, it could be useful to translate "cognitive structure" into behavioral terms for the purpose of devising methods of change.

In addition to the polarizations referred to in the previous section, the characteristics of contingency-shaped behavior and those of cognitive structures are similar in other ways. First, the effects of reinforcement occur at an unconscious level and structures are also unconscious. Second, the effects of reinforcement are functionally defined (i.e., behaviors different in appearance can achieve the same effect), which is consistent with the deep meaning attributed to cognitive structures. Third, reinforced behavior is changed through experience with contingencies and not through "talking about the contingencies," which corresponds to the nonessential presence of metacognition in changing cognitive structures.

Thus, we are suggesting that the core structures referred to by cognitive therapists are the same as contingency-shaped behaviors, which would mean that cognitive therapists should direct more attention to contingencies when they are attempting to change core structures. Paying attention to contingencies is exactly what Jacobson (1989) did when he described how he used the therapist-client relationship to change a client's core belief about her "badness." According to Jacobson, the core structure was changed by the client's taking "the risk of being known intimately" to him, and the client's risk being "paid off" in his continued acceptance and positive regard.

A conceptual difference between contingency-shaped behavior and cognitive structures is that the former is a behavioral entity and the latter is a nonbehavioral entity. Viewing structures as nonbehavioral entities has the unfortunate effect of distracting attention from behavioral processes. For example, cognitive therapists often do not recognize that the role of reinforcement is an inherent part of their procedures. The effect of a therapist's attention or the reactions of significant others can significantly impact what a client says or does. Regardless of one's theoretical orientation, it is accepted that reinforcement is a factor to be considered at least some of the time. Yet cognitive therapists in their theoretical analyses seem to have a phobia concerning the term *reinforcement*. Hollon and Kriss (1984) did not even make a passing reference to it. Similarly, in the foregoing case described by Jacobson (1989), the operations of reinforcement were described but the term *reinforcement* was not used. Even Wessells (1982), in an elegant defense of cognitive psychology, lamented that cognitivists, unfortunately, have neglected the role of contingencies in explaining behavior.

The neglect of the role of contingencies probably would occur in cognitive therapists' analysis of Harriet. From their perspective, Harriet's acquiescence would have occurred because of her underlying cognitive structures, and the structures are seen as entities that have existence independent of behavior. Given these assumptions, the cognitivists' account of Harriet's actions and methods of changing them would require something other than how one would directly account for and change a behavior. Needless to say, the FAP account of Harriet's actions involves behavior and clinical interventions that are described in terms of behavior change.

CLINICAL IMPLICATIONS OF THE FAP VIEW OF BELIEFS

Although we agree with cognitive therapists that thinking can precede actions, we regard the thought-behavior relationship always as a behavior-behavior relationship. When thoughts are considered as behavior, the therapist is led to consider the various origins of the thinking behaviors involved and, in particular, to pay attention to the ongoing contingencies of reinforcement in their development and modification. The four major implications of treating Bs as behavior are discussed below.

Focus on Thinking in the Here and Now

The client's thinking will be most subject to therapeutic change if it occurs close in time and place to relevant contingencies and stimulus control. Thus, whenever possible, we recommend focusing on thinking, believing, and other relevant behaviors that occur during the session. Opportunities to directly shape more adaptive Bs frequently occur as the client's dysfunctional thinking is brought into the client-therapist relationship. For example, assume that Harriet's problem is of the $A \rightarrow B$ $\rightarrow C$ variety. Then, Harriet's acquiescing occurs *because* she thought it showed how much she cares, and *because* she thought doing otherwise would have evoked the therapist's anger. These are examples of Bs occurring within the context of the relationship. Harriet's thinking could have been challenged and reinterpreted on the spot, and new behavior could have been encouraged.

In contrast to this position, cognitive therapists focus on behavior that occurs elsewhere. When this position is taken to its extreme, the cognitive therapist may explicitly avoid or prevent therapeutic opportunities provided by the therapist-client interaction. For example, in a discussion of "technical problems" in doing cognitive therapy for depression, Beck *et al.* (1979) raised the problem of a client who says, "You are more interested in doing research than in helping me." First, Beck wisely pointed out that even if nothing is said, a client who is in a clinical research project may be secretly harboring such thoughts. However, the reason such thoughts occur, according to Beck, is that depressed clients may be distorting what the therapist does. He then suggested that the therapist inquire if any such notions are present and then to put these worries to rest. According to Beck, if possible, the therapist should avoid such problems in the first place by anticipating their occurrence and giving complete explanations to the client.

A FAP analysis of that situation would be somewhat different. A depressed client who feels unimportant to the therapist highlights the fact that the therapy situation could be evoking the problem that the client experiences in daily life relationships—that of not acting as though she were important and asking for what she wants. This would be viewed as, not a technical problem to be disposed of, but a situation that provides an important therapeutic opportunity. Also, the FAP therapist would not assume that the client is distorting, just that the therapist is contacting different aspects of the current situation than the client. It is even possible that the research is more important to the therapist and, if so, the client would not be "distorting." The notion that the client might be secretly harboring such ideas rather than telling the therapist about them is also suggestive of the occurrence of the clinical problem of the client not being direct or assertive during the session.

Although his theory may, in general, lead the cognitive therapist to overlook situations that would be of interest to a FAP therapist, Beck recognized that certain therapist-client interactions can provide therapeutic opportunity. For example, in discussing ways to strengthen collaboration, he pointed out that a client may react to a homework assignment as a test of self-worth and that the therapist should try to sense this (Rule 1) and use it as an opportunity to correct faulty cognitions. Beck, however, gave no special significance to the fact that the therapeutic work focused on behavior as it is occurring. Instead, he viewed it as having the same effects as dealing with a cognition that occurs elsewhere. Jacobson (1989), on the other hand, discussed the importance of focusing on behavior during the session when doing Beck's cognitive therapy. Furthermore, he suggested that this factor be incorporated in the conceptual underpinnings of cognitive therapy for depression.

Take into Account the Varying Role That Thoughts Can Play

In addition to viewing thoughts as behavior, we believe that it is possible to have Bs that may or may not play a role in the client's problem. Recalling our previous discussion, we examined three possibilities: (1) that thought influences subsequent behavior; (2) that thought does not influence subsequent behavior; and (3) that thought contributes to the strength of a contingency-shaped subsequent behavior. In other words, the degree of control exerted by thinking over clinical symptoms is on a continuum. At one end is the pure $A \rightarrow B \rightarrow C$ type where the preceding B is a behavior that corresponds to a cognitive product and has an influence on the client's problem. Treatment for this type is aimed at changing Bs. The procedures outlined in Rule 5 for making interpretations are appropriate here and include the cognitive therapy techniques of logical arguments, questioning the evidence, and direct instructions to change beliefs.

At the other end of the continuum is the $A \rightarrow C$ type in which the symptom has been shaped purely by contingencies. In this case, treatment is aimed at directly changing the Cs—the focus would be on exposing the client to positive reinforcement in the therapy session and in the natural environment that would shape and sustain new Cs. The interpretations given to clients also would correspond to $A \rightarrow C$. To illustrate, take the case of Christina, who was raised by a paranoid schizophrenic mother and sexually abused by surrogate parents as a teenager. Even before she acquired language she was neglected, deprived, abused, and rejected, which continued throughout her childhood. Not surprisingly, she was frequently depressed and angry.

The excerpt that follows is from a session with Christina after she had been in treatment with the second author for 6 years:

C: Life is a vaudeville of horrors. I feel such a sense of humiliation. I don't want to struggle, I just want to figure out how to die. That's how I feel when I'm depressed. The only thing that would give me perspective is having someone in my life. Things don't seem as scary then. (It appears that the client is making an *ABC* interpretation of "I get depressed when I don't have anyone in my life" and "Right now, I don't have anyone, therefore I am depressed.")

T: You seem closed to me right now, you're not taking in my love and caring. (I responded as though the depression was an *ABC* problem by offering the interpretation that "I am in your life. All you have to do is accept that and then you won't be depressed.")

C: Your problem is you don't have any empathy. You've never been depressed the way that I am. If so, you wouldn't say things like "be open to me" and that your love should make things better. I'm alone 99% of the time, day after day, weekend after weekend, and you expect me to come in here and be an open little flower? (Christina is letting me know in no uncertain terms that she didn't like the *ABC* interpretation. It may have been similar to the invalidating demands made by others that she feel and act in ways that were convenient to them. See Chapter 6 on development of the self.)

In the foregoing example, making any type of interpretation that conveyed a demand to do or feel a certain way made Christina angry and was seen as unempathetic. I was in a difficult situation. Interpretations are a primary way that a therapist indicates that the client's ideas are taken seriously. In that vein, I wanted to make an interpretation that was consistent with her experience; that is, an $A \rightarrow C$ formulation, and at the same time, one that related Christina's response to me in the context of her history (Rule 5). Yet, it also needed to be empathic—free of demands so, I wrote her a poem:

Depression

Ravaged and depleted
by life's atrocities
drowning in my shame
trapped in a damp dark cave
with no hope for escape
a baby screaming inside
dying to be held
dying.

I reach out
but you do not hear me.
You and I are separated

by thick walls of glass.
You see me but cannot feel
the poison in my soul.
You talk to me about ways to get out
        of my prison,
but don't you see I need you
to be on my side
of the bars?

I have always been alone.
Alone as an infant,
battered by my mother's
depression and schizophrenia.
Alone as a child,
with no one to hold my hand.
Alone as an adolescent,
used as sex object
by surrogate parents and their friends.
Used . . . and discarded.

I desperately try to fill my emptiness
with faceless penises
which only slash at my heart.
Occasional glimpses of sunshine
through the layers of shit in my brain
are not enough . . .
I do not want to live.

I unleash my fury at you
because there is no one else.
But there is not even you.

I mailed the poem to her with this note: "Christina, I do not know how to reach you when you are depressed. This poem is an attempt to connect with you, to see the world through your eyes. I love you dearly. Hang on." She responded by telling me that it was one of the nicest things anyone had ever done for her.

During her childhood, Christina was treated as worthless; that is, she developed contingency-shaped behavior for taking care of others even though it damaged her (this is behavior that is consistent with the notion that she herself was worthless). She felt, acted, and described herself as worthless. According to our model, she self-tacted "I am worthless" ($A \rightarrow C \rightarrow B$). I accepted her thoughts of worthlessness as self-tacts which corresponded to her past and to her experience of herself. Thus, I did not use logic to convince Christina that her belief was incorrect and thereby to change her into a "worthwhile" person, especially since she knew all the logical arguments already. Nor did I treat Christina's self-worthlessness as a hypothesis that needed to be tested and rejected. Instead I focused on strengthening those repertoires that are characteristic of a "worthwhile" person. This procedure entailed reacting to her as a "worthwhile" person over a long period of time by seriously considering and reacting to all of her thoughts and ideas, by treating her with caring and respect, by putting in the time and energy that are due to a worthwhile person. The poem was consistent with this approach.

Needless to say, treating Christina's experience of depression and worthlessness as "irrational" would have been countertherapeutic because of the implicit rejection and belittling of her thoughts and feelings. Thus, from a behavioral standpoint, the appropriate therapy for a client with this type of $A \rightarrow C$ problem is more like the "corrective emotional experience" advocated by some psychodynamically oriented therapists.

Offer Relevant Explanations of Client Problems

Our analysis also has implications for explanations offered to clients about their problems. Although it is possible for a client with an $A \rightarrow C$ problem to improve when given an $A \rightarrow B \rightarrow C$ interpretation, less favorable outcomes are also possible. This is especially true for clients who grew up in dysfunctional families with adults who were not sensitive to their feelings. Many of our clients suffered emotional abuse, including neglect, negation, or punishment for their expression of feelings. Children who are repeatedly told, either directly or indirectly, that "there's no reason for you to feel or think that way" often grow up with problems of the self (see Chapter 6 for elaboration). They do not trust their feelings and are unsure of who they are. Treating such clients with cognitive therapy techniques and giving them explanations which suggest that their assumptions, beliefs, or attitudes are dysfunctional and/or irrational contain the risk of replaying the contingencies that are associated with the invalidation and alienation they experienced while growing up. Additionally, $A \rightarrow C$ clients who are treated as though their problem were $A \rightarrow B \rightarrow C$, might drop out of treatment if they feel invalidated and alienated.

Another possibility is that clients who are incorrectly told that their problems are controlled by preceding thoughts and not by a reinforcement history may spend too much time working on their thoughts to the exclusion of experiencing the real world. For example, take the case of a woman whose fears of rejection stem from early preverbal experiences with a psychotic mother. Her reactions to rejection are immediate and unconscious. It is more important for this client to be exposed to a variety of interpersonal experiences that are not followed by the extreme consequences she experienced with her mother than to be engaged in lengthy logical arguments about giving up the irrational idea "I need to be loved by everyone all the time."

Use Direct Cognitive Manipulation with Caution

We have been focusing on the problems that can occur when treating an $A \rightarrow C$ problem as though it were an $A \rightarrow B \rightarrow C$ problem. Nevertheless, the direct cognitive manipulations sometimes used by cognitive therapists can benefit clients even if their problem is mainly an $A \rightarrow C$ type. We define direct cognitive manipulation as therapist behaviors that involve appeals to reason, logical arguments, or telling the client that a particular belief does not match the therapist's observations. Thus, direct cognitive manipulation is primarily rule-giving. When the client responds to the rule by changing their Bs (cognitive products such as beliefs and automatic thoughts), these changes are rule-governed behavior. This process can be of benefit to the client for several reasons. First, it seems reasonable to posit that beliefs contribute, at least to some degree, to many client problems even if the primary factor is the result of contingencies. This paradigm is illustrated in Figure 2c. Cognitive therapy methods aimed at directly changing B then would be helpful, particularly if the client also were exposed to contingencies for improved behavior.

Cognitive therapy techniques for $A \rightarrow C$ problems also might benefit some clients who are linear and logical thinkers and who already interpret their problem according to the ABC hypothesis (even though their problem is $A \rightarrow C$). The benefit occurs because such persons have learned to be consistent. That is, they grew up in environments where "practicing what you preach" was highly valued and "saying one thing and doing another" was not. There is some inclination for this type of client to act in accordance with a "belief" that a therapist has directly instructed a client to hold. The strength of such inclinations, however, is generally weak and is dependent on how much emphasis was placed on consistency in the client's subculture.

Another way direct cognitive manipulation can help with $A \rightarrow C$ problems is through the covert contingencies and rules that such procedures engender. For example, an unintended effect of rationally convincing clients to hold a certain belief is that it involves a therapist demand or description that implies that if the clients behave as told they will get better (a rule). If the clients then behave differently, and this new way of behaving is naturally reinforced, the clients improve.

For instance, convincing Harriet that she *can* stand anger could be viewed as a therapist's covert demand or implied instruction for her to act differently. Changes in Harriet's behavior would then be the result of her following instructions or rule-governed behavior. Significant clinical improvement will occur if her new behavior is naturally reinforced in her daily life. This process is more obvious when the cognitive therapy involves explicit, overt instructions to the client for behavior change. For example, Beck *et al.* (1979) encouraged clients to act against their assumptions because it is "the most powerful way to change it" (p. 264). Although Beck preferred to view this intervention as changing a cognition (an assumption), it can also be seen as the therapist's issuing a rule, and the client's following a rule that results in exposing the client's behavior to contingencies which directly strengthen the improved behavior. This emphasis on building in new behavior is consistent with FAP.

However, when cognitive products and subsequent behavior change because the client is trying please the therapist, it can be countertherapeutic. The danger is that the improvements will not be maintained by the natural reinforcers in the client's daily life and the gains made in therapy will be lost when therapy ends. This problem was discussed in Chapter 2 under the topic of arbitrary versus natural reinforcement. Since direct cognitive manipulations involve direct instructions on how to think or behave and make explicit demands for improvements, it is difficult to avoid pleasing the therapist. A notable exception is Beck *et al.*'s (1979) use of the Socratic method and "hypothesis testing" which we view as ingenious ways of reducing motivation to please the therapist and of bringing clients into contact with natural reinforcers.

Although FAP therapists may use appeals to reason, theoretical differences between FAP and cognitive therapies lead to different therapist behaviors when such interventions are not successful. One approach that the cognitive therapist might try would be to come up with additional arguments as to why the client's thoughts are incorrect. From a FAP perspective, getting Harriet to change her belief by rationally convincing her, (à la Albert Ellis) that "she *can* stand anger" is not guaranteed to have a favorable result when she actually finds herself in the problem situation in the future. No guarantee exists, because it is unclear what behavior has been changed due to the "convincing," other than her saying, "Okay, I believe I can stand it."

When the client changes a belief statement because of the logical arguments of the therapist, the meaning of the statement changes. Before the therapeutic intervention, the belief statement had the property of being a description of past experiences or indication of the likelihood of certain actions. After the client's beliefs are changed on account of to the therapist's logical argument, it is no longer derived from experience but is instead a response made to please the therapist or to conform to the rules of logic. It is therefore not surprising that many clients who have been "convinced" to change their beliefs subsequently do not change their behavior in the problem situation. Such "failures" are usually accompanied by explanations such as "I intellectually believe it, but I don't accept it on an emotional level." The FAP therapist would not find this state of affairs perplexing since there is no reason to expect anything else.

In contrast, we would instead accept the client's "inconsistencies" and try to identify variables that account for behaviors, such as (1) espousing belief X and acting consistent with belief Y, (2) trying to be consistent in espousing and acting, or (3) trying to please the therapist by being rational.

CASE ILLUSTRATION

In the case of Kelly (first described in Chapter 4) the B seemed to contribute to the strength of her contingency-shaped behavior. Her treatment and an explanation of her behavior was based on this model. Kelly had chaotic relationships with men partly because of her erratic actions, and was about to recreate the same pattern by prematurely ending therapy with the first author. When asked why she wanted to quit, Kelly said she was doing this *because* she was getting the feeling that I was, in fact, about to tell her that I was not going to see her anymore, and she thought she should end it first. Although this sounds like a pure $A \rightarrow B \rightarrow C$ problem in which the B was her hypothesis about my intentions, I assumed that contingency-shaped behavior was also present because Kelly could not identify anything that I did to give her this impression. This is the phenomenon that leads psychodynamic therapists to say that the causes of Kelly's avoidance were unconscious.

Kelly's history of abandonment, dating back to childhood, and her avoidance of the possibility of further abandonment by withdrawing from close relationships also supported the hypothesis of the presence of contingency-shaped behavior.

Thus, the occurrence of the CRB1 of prematurely ending therapy was used as an *in vivo* opportunity for Kelly to check out her assumptions. I reassured her that I was committed to completing the therapy and would not precipitously end it. Thus assured, Kelly's fears were assuaged and she remained in therapy. Since her problem was also contingency-shaped, the reassurances only had temporary effects and her fears would return. At times, however, she could think about my reassurance and thereby moderate her avoidance behavior and emotional reactions.

I offered Kelly an interpretation based on the combined effects of a conscious *B* and an unconscious contingency-shaped behavior. I explained how telling herself that "He hasn't abandoned me yet, and there's no evidence he will, and he said he wouldn't" could produce the same beneficial effects as my telling her the same thing. I also pointed out, however, that she had past experiences in which she was abandoned under similar conditions to the therapy, and that these were unconscious and not mediated by her self-statements. At times, therefore, she would experience fear and try to avoid me even if she tried to consciously reassure herself. She felt this interpretation corresponded to her feelings. As the therapeutic relationship evolved, the contingencies were present to reinforce behavior that was consistent with her thoughts that I would not abandon her. For example, I was consistent in keeping appointments, and when holidays or travel disrupted the schedule, I tried to schedule makeup sessions. The new, improved *B* (such as "It doesn't seem like he will abandon me") thus helped to develop the contingency-shaped behavior of "hanging in there to give it a chance" and vice versa.

In summary, we have presented a model in which thoughts either do, do not, or partially contribute to clinical problems. Although this model accommodates cognitive therapy techniques, it emphasizes the importance of contingencies in determining or altering the effects of thinking on other behavior. Thus, the use of appeals to rationality in FAP are only one small part of a larger set of therapeutic interactions that will help to develop a new set of client experiences and behaviors, and to produce a favorable change in associated believing.

6

The Self

Undoubtedly there is a familiar ring in the following interaction between Beatrice and her therapist:

Beatrice: It's so fucking hard to be real, to be me.

Therapist: If you aren't you, who are you?

Beatrice: I'm whoever someone else wants me to be. I don't even know when I'm being myself.

The "self" that Beatrice is talking about possesses some perplexing attributes. First, she is referring to her self as something different from her body; that is, she is describing her self as changing with other people's wants even though her body obviously remains the same. Her self, then, is not physical—it is not her body. Second, she implies that there is an inner experience of self that is controlled by external others. And, finally, she states that this self that she experiences is not really her *because* it is controlled by others. This, in turn, implies that there is or could be an experience of her real self which is unchanging and not controlled by others.

Such paradoxes abound when one looks at the literature on the self. These perplexities have invoked one author to title his treatise on the self, "Is Anyone in Charge?" (Greenwald, 1982). In this chapter, we will provide a behavioral conception of self that accounts for these paradoxes and several "normal" or typical senses of the self as well as "pathological" states or problems of the self. We will then show how to apply our behavioral model to treatment.

We will begin by scoping out the dimensions of the self that will be included in our account. Our model will explain, in behavioral terms,

125

the essential features of these nonpathological descriptions as well the pathological descriptions of self.

COMMON DEFINITIONS OF THE SELF

The four descriptions of the self by nonbehaviorists that follow represent common, everyday, nonpathological usages of the term:

1. *Experience of the self as the "I."* Most of us have an "I" feeling. According to Deikman (1973), this "I" is "an abiding, resting awareness, featureless and unchanging, a central something that is witness to all events, exterior and interior" (p. 325). Deikman also described this self as identical to awareness.

2. *The self as an originator of action*. Another type of "I" that is felt is the one in "I want," such as "I want a new car" or "I will not get up from my typewriter until this paper is done." Deikman described this "I" as the organizing force compelling the individual to act.

3. *The self as a source of spontaneous gestures*. According to Winnicott (1965), the "real" or "true" self is the source of spontaneous gestures and personal ideas. Similarly, Masterson (1985) viewed creativity as "the ultimate of real self expression" (p. 17). The false self, on the other hand, does not have original ideas but only has ideas that come from others.

4. *The self as personal identity*. Erikson (1968) described personal identity as the conscious experience of two simultaneous perceptions: (a) selfsameness—"the perception of the selfsameness and continuity of one's existence in time and space," and (b) other recognition of selfsameness— "the perception of the fact that others recognize one's sameness and continuity" (p. 50).

These descriptions represent common notions about the self in both clinical practice and in everyday experience. The concepts which are used in describing the self seem outside of the behavioral realm, and a behaviorist who attempts to explain these phenomena encounters considerable obstacles. For example, how does one specify in behavioral terms such notions as "knowing what one wants," "not being me," or "a featureless and unchanging awareness"?

The very notion of a "self" as an explanatory concept is antithetical to the behaviorist's avoidance of internal entities to explain behavior.

When one attempts to explain client behavior in terms of problems of the self (where the self is a nonbehavioral entity), a homuncular fictional entity has been reified and then erroneously used to explain behavior. For example, one could say that the extreme dependence of a client on the therapist is caused by an inadequate self. That is, the therapist makes up for this inadequacy by providing a more complete self; hence the client becomes dependent because he or she experiences a more adequate self with the therapist. This type of explanation is not satisfying to the behaviorist because "complete self" and "inadequate self" are new, nonbehavioral structures that still need to be accounted for. Not wanting to resort to these types of misleading explanations, behaviorists, in general, have avoided using the term and correspondingly have not focused on problems of the self or treatment thereof.

To date, the only exception has been Skinner, who has made a number of theoretical analyses of the self (1953, 1957) and has laid the groundwork for a more complete behavioral account. Our intention is to develop Skinner's notions and explore the clinical implications. There are at least two reasons why such an endeavor should be undertaken. First, client problems that are described in terms of self disorders appear to be important and prevalent. One indication of this is found in the burgeoning literature devoted to the topic within modern psychoanalysis, self-psychology, and object relations. Second, the phenomenon of self seems to be part of the human experience, and clients often describe their problems in terms of their self.

A BEHAVIORAL FORMULATION OF SELF

Any adequate explanation of the self would have to account for the experience or sense of self. This is true because so many of the descriptions of normal and pathological self involve the experience of the person (e.g., "experiencing a continuity and selfsameness" or the clients who "do not know who they are"). Accordingly, our account is aimed at understanding and explaining the sense or experience of self. Although ideas differ as to what constitutes an explanation or understanding of an experience, we feel it is advantageous to understand what is experienced by identifying the stimuli that evoke the feeling or sensation and the kind of previous experiences that affect this process. Although this approach might appear esoteric when stated in formal terms, it is a commonly used method in everyday experience.

To illustrate, suppose we are trying to understand a person's experience of being hot. We could put a person in a temperature-controlled room, vary the temperature, record body temperature, and find out what temperature is required for the person to report "I'm hot." By varying the humidity, we would similarly derive the contribution of this variable to the experience. Our understanding would be even greater, however, if we could find out more about this person's previous experience with heat. If he or she grew up in the desert, for example, a considerable increase in room temperature might be required to evoke the "hot" response than required for someone who was born and raised in Alaska. This approach to explanation involves knowing more about the factors related to the experience. More specifically, the more we know about the variables that result in the person's reporting "hot," the more we can say we "understand" his or her experience. As you may have noted, our approach to understanding a person's experience is intimately connected to understanding the verbal report of that experience. Although they are not the same, we are assuming that the same factors that affect one's experience also affect the verbal report of that experience. Some readers may object to this equivalence on the basis that their own experience is nonverbal. We ask these readers to reserve their final judgment on this issue. A nonverbal experience of self is consistent with the present behavioral analysis.

Our approach to understanding the experience of self parallels that of heat. Just as we would explain the experience of heat by identifying the stimulus and history for the response "I feel hot," we will try to explain the experience of self by describing the stimuli and history that account for the words that identify the self. These words include "I," "me," "Baby," "Davie" or "Dottie" (when used to refer to one's self), and "you" (when used by a young child to refer to one's self). For illustrative purposes, however, we will confine our discussion to the generic "I." Our approach to the understanding of "I," with some slight variations, would apply as well to "I" synonyms and other equivalents. Thus, our analysis of "I" can be viewed as a prototype for the analysis of other verbal responses associated with the self. As it turns out, an understanding of "I" in particular does seem to account for a wide range of experiences of self. Specification of the stimuli for "I" also illuminates the nature of the stimulus that in general controls the experience of self.

Basic Concepts

Our hypothesis about self is essentially a hypothesis about verbal behavior. Specifically, it is that understanding the experience of self is the specification of the stimuli controlling the verbal response "I." Several verbal behavior concepts form the foundation of our approach: *stimulus control*, *tact*, *functional units*, and the *emergence of small functional units*. Since stimulus control and tacts have already been discussed, only a brief review will be offered.

Stimulus Control

Imagine a pigeon who is reinforced for pecking a key only when a signal light is illuminated. Eventually, the illumination of the signal will be followed by a key-peck response. Some obvious statements we could make about this situation are:

1. The response, pecking the key, occurs when the Sd (discriminative stimulus—the illuminated signal light) is present.
2. Pecking the key is under the stimulus control of the signal light.
3. Pecking the key is a functional unit, defined as the behavior that occurs between the Sd and the reinforcer. (We will discuss this in more detail in the section on functional units.)

Because it will be important in understanding our behavioral conception of self, we are going to elaborate on the process by which the signal light becomes an Sd. At the beginning of the experiment, the pigeon is actually exposed to a broad stimulus array consisting of the signal light, movements and noises in the environment, room lights, the pigeon's own orienting to the light, as well as a wealth of internal or private stimuli such as physiological activity and kinesthetic stimulation from orienting to the signal light. Thus, even though the experimenter may feel that the signal light is the most obvious stimulus, it is not necessarily so to the pigeon. With repeated trials, however, the signal light does become salient enough to control the key-peck response because it is the one stimulus element in the complex stimulus array that is always present when reinforcers are delivered.

The Tact

Imagine a baby girl who is just learning how to talk, and is reinforced by her parent's joy for saying "apple" only when an apple is shown, and not when a banana or an orange is shown. Eventually, just having the apple present will result in the child's saying "apple" or "appee" or "ahp" as the case may be. Some obvious statements we could make about this situation are:

1. The response, the utterance "apple," occurs when the Sd (discriminative stimulus), an apple, is present.
2. The response "apple" is under the stimulus control of the apple.
3. The response "apple" is a functional unit.
4. We would not say that the tact *apple* stands for an apple any more than we would say that the key pecking in the pigeon experiment stands for the signal light. Correspondingly, we would not say the child uses the word *apple* any more than we would say the pigeon uses the key peck.

Just as in the case of the pigeon and the signal light, the actual apple came to control the response "apple" because it was the one stimulus that was present each time saying "apple" was reinforced. Although obvious, in order for this verbal conditioning to take place, the parent had to see the apple (i.e., know it was present). As we will point out later on, the importance of the parent knowing that the Sd is present is a major issue when the child is learning "I."

Functional Units

As previously pointed out, the pigeon's key peck is a functional unit. When we see a peck occurring, we can say, "That's one." When it comes to verbal behavior, however, it is less clear what is counted as a unit or a single occurrence. Even though it is tempting to say the unit of verbal behavior is a word, this quickly leads to problems, however, because we experience our utterances as being sometimes larger and sometimes smaller than a word. One example comes from when the first author first learned the national anthem. I remember learning one large senseless unit—"landaliverty." Similarly, the alphabet is usually learned in larger units as evidenced by the difficulty in starting at some random point. Conversely, some complex words, such as dihydroergotamine, may be really a combination of smaller units "di," "hydro," and "ergotamine."

The functional unit is Skinner's conception of the unit of verbal behavior and its size depends on how it was learned and maintained. Since a functional unit is the behavior that occurs between the Sd and the reinforcer, the actual size of the unit can change with experience. For example, a young child might first be prompted to say "baby" as two smaller units—the parent says "bay," waits for the child to say "bay," and then the parent says "good and now say bee." After this type of prompting, when the child is asked to tact a baby, he or she might say a word like "bay-bee," which still evidences the two smaller units from which it was composed. In time, however, a single unit "baby" will emerge. Thus, functional units can be small in size like words ("apple" and "boy") and phonemes ("bay" and "bee"). Larger units of verbal behavior would be phrases like "How are you," "God save the Queen," "ice cream," and "The United States of America." Even larger units, like the Pledge of Allegiance and the Gettysburg Address, if recited as a whole, include the alphabet.

The Emergence of Small Functional Units

For the purposes of this chapter, we are particularly interested in "I" as a small functional unit; that is, as an individual word which has independent meaning. We are going to contrast two ways a single word can become a functional unit when a child is learning to talk. This single-word functional unit can be separately learned, or it can emerge as a by-product of the acquisition of larger responses containing identical elements (Skinner, 1957, p. 120). Separate learning of a word as a unit was illustrated in the previous example, which showed how the tact "apple" was acquired. In that example, the word *apple* was learned as a unit.

Now we will use an example to explain how a word can become a unit via emergence from the acquisition of larger units. The word *big* is used in our illustration. Let's assume that a little boy has the tacts "apple," "truck," "pencil," "orange," and "dog," but not "big" in his repertoire. His parent then points to a large apple in a bowl of apples and says, "That's a big apple; say 'big apple.'" After a number of such experiences and after the prompt has been faded, the boy will tact a large apple as "bigapple." Note that at this point, because of specific conditions under which the child is learning, "big" is not a functional unit. In fact, "bigapple" is a single unit without any connection to apple and thus is not a combination of the two units "big" and "apple". Next the parent prompts "big truck." Following a number of experiences with the large truck, the child tacts "bigtruck." Eventually, after the child has had a sufficient number of similar experiences with large oranges, dolls, pencils, and the like, the word *big* emerges as a small unit controlled by the stimulus of relative size. This happens because "big" is the identical element across a variety of situations in which the specific objects (oranges, dolls, pencils) vary, and largeness is a common stimulus element. After the unit "big" has emerged, the child will then be able to tact "big dog" even though he never has had any previous experience with large dogs.

In contrast to the process in which "big" emerges from larger units, it would have been possible to arrange learning experiences so that "big" was separately acquired. To do so, the parent would point at the large apple and prompt "big" (rather than "big apple") so that the child tacts "big." The same is repeated for other objects until largeness comes to control "big."

The above examples are intended to illustrate two methods by which a word can become a functional unit. We have purposely simplified the learning experiences and described them in a stereotyped way in order to clarify the role of the fundamental processes that are involved. We are not suggesting that our examples precisely correspond to how a child learns "big" in the natural environment. In real life, prompts, modeling, and reinforcement are used more haphazardly and inconsistently. Thus, the word *big* is probably acquired through a combination of separate learning and emergence from larger units and/or other processes less relevant to our discussion (e.g., learning meaning through definition).

As a child is learning to talk, he or she simultaneously acquires single functional units ranging in size from small to large. The period of life between 6 months and 2 years is known as the "single-word speech period" to linguists and developmental psychologists. We believe it would be more accurate to call this the "single functional unit period" because the child might learn units that are larger or smaller than a word but yet are still a single functional unit. Observations of children's language during this period supports the functional unit view (Dore, 1985). At the beginning of this period, the single units are words or fragments of words, such as "doll," "apple," "app" (for apple), "crea" (for ice cream), "down" (for fall down). Toward the end of this period or the second year of life, many of these *single words* have the form of two- or three-word phrases like as "bite-you," "baby-bite-you," "more-juice," and "I-more-juice" but are still functionally single units. At this young age, the larger units are not composed by the child from smaller units; they are learned as a whole.

The Emergence of "I" as a Small Functional Unit

We propose that "I"* emerges as a functional unit from the acquisition of larger units as a child learns to speak during normal, non-pathological, development. We have designated three developmental stages relevant to this emergence and have illustrated them in Figure 4,

---

*Our analysis of the term "I" also applies to "mine," "my," "me," "proper name," and the like, and it is assumed these terms overlap in functional meaning.

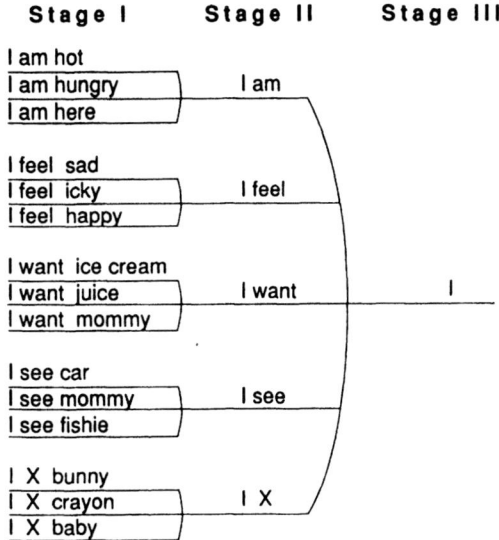

Figure 4. The three stages of verbal behavior development that result in "I" emerging as a small functional unit. In Stage I, the child learns larger independent units that are the basis of the more abstract intermediate-sized units of Stage II. Then, the "I" of Stage III emerges from the medium-sized units of Stage II.

which shows units of three sizes, with each corresponding to a developmental stage.

During Stage I, the child learns numerous large units, such as "I have a doll," "I have a bunny," "I want ice cream," "I want juice," "I see the car," and "I see mommy." Keep in mind that the real life form of these might be "me see mama" or "baby ice cream," and that we are using "I" as a generic form of self-reference. These large units are learned as a whole (i.e., they are functional units). This stage occurs during the first 2 years of life.

During Stage II, smaller functional units emerge, such as "I have," "I want," and "I see," which can then be combined with particular objects. It is during this stage that a child can say, "I want football" even though she or he may never have uttered this particular phrase before.

During Stage III, a single, even smaller unit "I" emerges, and at the same time, the experience of "I." From our perspective, the acquisition of the experience of "I" is similar to one's acquisition of the experience of a football, ice cream, mommy, or heat in that they are all tacts. These experiences differ from "I," however, in that they are under the control of specific public stimuli and can be separately learned. "I," on the other hand, is under the control of a complex private stimulus and appears to be almost exclusively learned through its emergence from larger units.

The real understanding of the self-experience comes from the description of the stimuli that control the responses in each of the three stages. As these functional units evolve into "I," there is a corresponding shift in the controlling stimuli and a greater emphasis on private components.

Stage I: Learning Large Functional Units

As in all discrimination learning, the parent* must use public stimuli (stimuli available to the parent) when teaching their children to tact. We have pointed out earlier the obvious fact that a parent must be able to see the apple, a public stimulus, in order to teach the tact "apple." Now look at the public stimulus a parent uses to help a child learn a similar but different tact, "I see apple," as a large unit. We are viewing the tacts "apple" and "I see apple" as having different meanings (e.g., being controlled by different stimuli in the normal adult speaker). The simple tact "apple" is controlled merely by the presence of the apple. In everyday terms, we would say the tact describes the external stimulus as in "that's an apple." The tact "I see apple," however, is controlled by an activity of the speaker—seeing. In everyday terms, it describes an *activity* of the speaker so we will refer to this activity as *seeing*. In some cases, the activity of seeing may have nothing to do with the presence of an external stimulus as when the speaker is imagining an apple (Skinner, 1957).

Now consider how the parent teaches the child to come under control of the activity of seeing when saying, "I see apple." In one way or another, the parent prompts and encourages the child to say, "I see apple," when it is apparent that the child is seeing the apple. The parent, however, cannot directly observe the child "seeing an apple" because this is private and is available only to the child. The question is, which public stimuli does the parent use to indirectly observe the child's seeing and then which stimuli actually come to control the child's response? Again, our description of this process is purposely stereotyped and simplified to clarify the basic learning processes that are involved. In real life, the parent teaches the child in a more casual and inconsistent manner although the fundamental processes are the same.

---

*We recognize that primary teachers of children include persons other than the parents. For simplicity, however, we use the term parent to refer to all those persons who participate in teaching the child.

The top portion of Figure 5 (a-c) shows a sample of public stimuli on the left and private stimuli on the right that are present when the parent prompts the child to say, "I see apple." Perspective (shown in Figure 5a) is the spatial relation between the child and external objects. Although it is a public stimulus that is present, it does not enter into the child's learning of "I see apple" at this time. (It is shown because it is discussed later.) The public stimuli shown in the left half of Figures 5b and 5c are those that the parent could potentially use to know whether the child is "seeing an apple." These public stimuli are the orienting of the child toward the apple and an apple itself. The orienting the parent observes could include head-turning, widening of the eyes, and intense staring in the general direction of the apple. The actual components of orienting would probably vary slightly from time to time.

In addition to these public stimuli, a wealth of additional private stimulation, accessible only to the child, is represented as the less distinct objects shown under the Private Stimuli column in the top part of Figure 5. One such stimulus would be the private activity associated with the public orienting toward the apple (right side of Figure 5b). This private component of orienting perhaps corresponds to the physiological components of the orienting reflex. Another would be the particular visual system activity associated with seeing the apple (right side of Figure 5c), as well as a general component that we have designated as "seeing" (Figure 5d). The general component of seeing is that which occurs regardless of what is being seen. The private components of perspective (right side of Figure 5a) are also present. Since we cannot access private stimuli, we can only hypothesize that there are many additional ones involving any form of internal activity, such as visual, auditory, olfactory, gustatory, autonomic, and kinesthetic stimuli.

In the simplified situation we are describing in which the parent is teaching, for the first time, the child to tact "I see apple," we can expect the essential public stimuli to gain control of the child's "I see apple." These are the very same stimuli that the parent uses to know if the child is seeing the apple. Thus, during this early stage of development, the tact, "I see apple," is learned as a unit and is controlled by the presence of the apple and the public aspects of orienting as shown in Figure 5e. Although private stimuli and other public stimuli (e.g., perspective) are present during the learning, they are not shown in Figure 5e because there is no reason for them to become Sd's and they have no effect. In this sense, they are irrelevant, not noticed, and thus not experienced. At this point in the development of the child, the statement, "I see apple," does not, as in an adult, involve a description of the experience of seeing. Instead, at this stage, "I see apple" probably has a meaning much closer

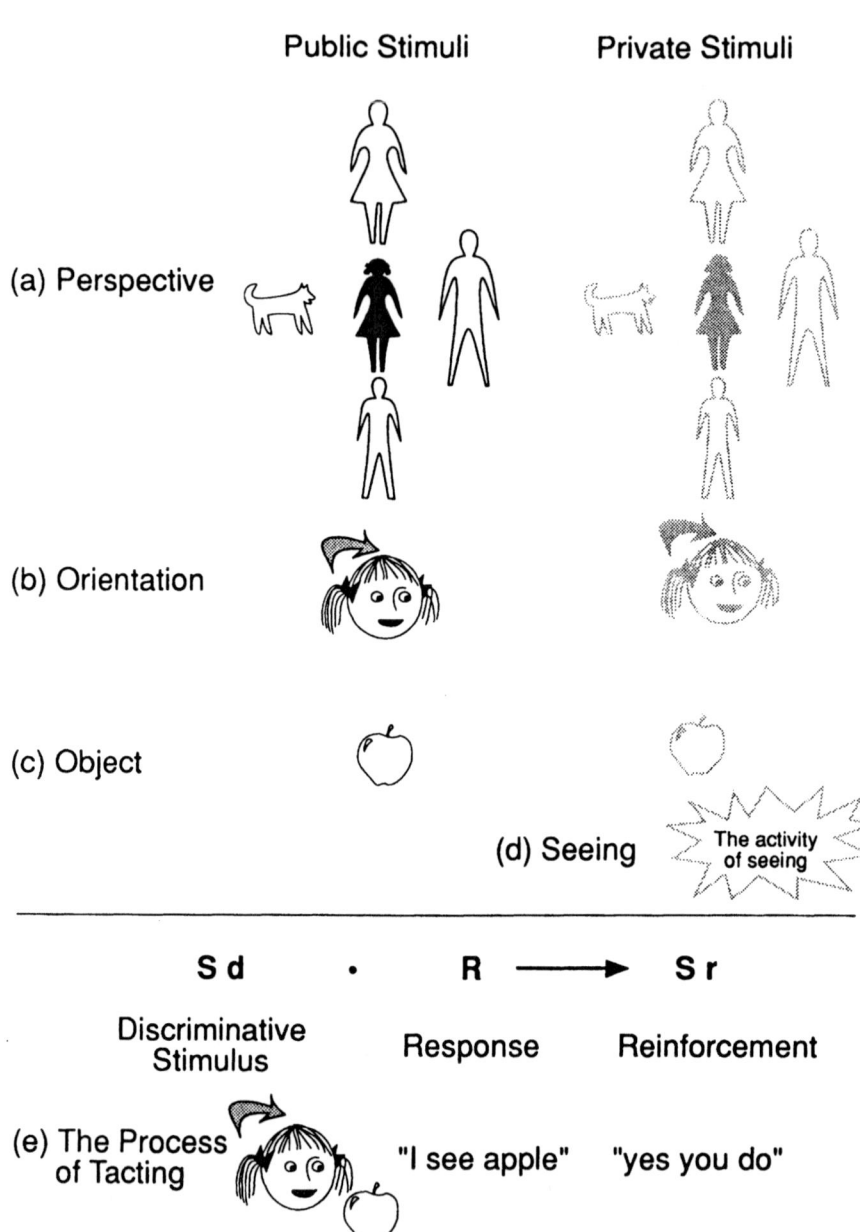

Public Stimuli   Private Stimuli

(a) Perspective

(b) Orientation

(c) Object

(d) Seeing   The activity
                    of seeing

S d   •   R ⟶   S r

Discriminative   Response   Reinforcement
Stimulus

(e) The Process   "I see apple"   "yes you do"
    of Tacting

Figure 5. In the top section, the public and private stimuli present when the child first learns to say "I see apple," including (a) the perspective that is the spatial relation between the child and external objects, (b) the orienting such as head-turning and widening of the eyes, (c) an apple, and (d) the private activity of seeing. In the bottom section, (e) shows that the discriminative stimuli, which come to control the response, are the public orienting and the apple.

to the simple tact "apple." Although the private stimuli do not play a role at this stage, they are important in later stages.

During Stage I, other large units involving "I" in addition to "I see apple" are also learned. "I want soy milk," "I am hot," and "I throw ball" are examples. Our discussion focuses on "I see," but the analysis applies to the other units as well.

Stage II: Learning Smaller Functional Units and the Development of Control by Private Stimuli

After learning a number of large functional units involving "I see," such as "I see a goat," "I see Daddy," and "I see doggy," the smaller functional unit "I see" of Stage II emerges. The smaller unit of "I see," once acquired, can now be combined with almost any other tact that is in the repertoire, and the child can now generate unique utterances. The "I see" emerges as a unit because it is an identical element in each of the varieties of "I see X" responses. The public orienting that the parent used to know that the child was seeing would be somewhat different in each of the various "I see" situations. For example, if the child were looking at an airplane in the sky, the orienting would be different than if looking at the parent's face. Although the stimulation from orienting would vary with the object being seen, the private stimuli associated with the activity of "seeing" is the same during all of the "I see X's" regardless of what "X" is. The private activity of seeing is shown in Figure 5d. It consistently is present only during "I see" situations and not "I want" or other "I" combinations. Therefore, it seems likely that the private stimulus associated with the activity of "seeing" would gain control of "I see."

If "I see" becomes controlled by private stimuli as we have suggested, then the "I see apple" response would have a different meaning than "That's an apple." The latter would be merely a description of the external stimulus or, in more precise terms, a tact controlled by the apple. The former, "I see apple," is now a combination of two smaller units where "apple" is a tact controlled by the external stimulus and "I see" is a tact controlled by the activity (seeing) of the speaker.

We are defining the ideal nonpathological environment as one that results in the control of "I see" and other intermediate-sized Stage II units (e.g., I want, I am, I feel, I have) by private stimuli. This type of environment would involve parents who prompt and reinforce the child for saying "I see X" whenever the child was in fact seeing the object X and not at other times when the child is seeing Y. This ideal is impossible to achieve, however, since parents cannot see inside the child and must rely on external signs. Thus, the parents' discriminative skill and attentiveness to these public stimuli are important factors in determining to what degree "I see" will be controlled by the private stimulus.

To illustrate, assume that "I see" has emerged as a functional unit during Stage II after considerable experience with many larger units, such as "I see ball," "I see kitty," and "I see car." At this point, both public and private stimuli are present that could control the response "I see." If the child then reports seeing an imagined stimulus as in the fantasizing or mental imaging that children do, then the child sees in the absence of the public stimuli with only private stimuli present. The parent who supports the validity of such experiences by taking the child's report seriously is reinforcing control by private stimuli. As a result, the child more likely will say "I see object X" based on his or her private seeing activity. The parent who ridicules or criticizes the child at this point will lessen control by private stimuli and the child more likely will say "I see object X" only when his or her public orienting responses and X are conspicuous (to the parent and thus to the child).

Keep in mind that we are not describing the process in which a child becomes reluctant to report his or her internal visual experiences because of fear or embarrassment. This type of suppression can occur only after the object is seen. We are describing the process by which the object is seen in the first place: the genesis of the relationship (or lack thereof) between internal experience and seeing.

Another important source of reinforcement of the control of "I see" by the private stimulation of "seeing" is the acceptance of the child's "I see" reports in situations where parents cannot see the public stimulus or it is obscure (e.g., a fish in the water which darts away after the child reports its presence, or a rabbit camouflaged in the foliage). Parents who take their children's "I see" reports seriously when the parent cannot see the controlling stimulus provide a normal or nonpathological environment whereby private stimuli eventually control the behavior. One indication of success in teaching private control of "I see" would be their child's ability to respond to a request to do imagery exercises. Other end results would be the ability to provide useful reports on threshold stimuli as used in psychophysics research or in the optometrist's exam. (The effects of unsuccessful training are discussed under pathological development.)

Stage III: The Development of "I" Through Private Stimuli

After a sufficient number of "I X" tacts have been learned, the child enters Stage III and the smaller unit "I" emerges. "I" is an identical element in each of the "I X" situations in which "X" varies.

Let us now turn to the stimuli that control "I." In normal development, "I" is a tact under the control of those stimuli that are common
to each of the "I X" tacts regardless of whether X is seeing, wanting,
having, and so forth. It is the same process by which "I see" emerged
as a unit under the stimulus control of "seeing" from "I see apple," "I
see truck," and the like.

We use the term *perspective*, mentioned earlier in our discussion and
shown in Figure 5a, to represent the stimulus which controls "I." We
have borrowed this term from Hayes (1984), who discussed the notion
of perspective in his radical behavioral analysis of spirituality. As shown
in Figure 5a, perspective has both public and private components and
includes the physical characteristics of the child's location in space in
relation to others. It is where the child is, right here, as opposed to where
the child is not—over there. In Figure 5a, the child is represented as the
darker, central figure and all other objects (people, dog, etc.) are located
with respect to the child. It is the public stimulus of perspective that
the parent uses to appropriately teach the child to tact "You want ice
cream" versus "I want ice cream" and "I see bunny" versus "You see
bunny." The public aspects of perspective are also involved when a parent is modeling the response, "I see a doll" while the child is conspicu-
ously looking at the doll. The parent is oriented to the child and/or
otherwise indicating who is supposed to say "I see a doll." If another
child is also present in the room, the parent acts in such a way that it
is clear which child is to say "I see a doll."

Perspective is the stimulus that remains constant for all the "I want
Xs," and "I see Xs," etc., since the Xs and the activities (wanting, seeing,
etc.) vary from time to time. The public aspects of the stimulus would
vary considerably with the particular situation. Sometimes the child may
be 5 feet to the left of the parent and at other times may be 50 feet
away. Given the wide variation in where "here" versus "there" may be,
a private aspect seems likely to gain control. During nonpathological
development, perspective is the physical location of the private activities
such as seeing, wanting, and having. Thus, the response "I" as a unit
is under the stimulus control of a locus.

Qualities of the "I" *freely describing wants & beliefs.*

As a means of showing the characteristics of the private stimulus
that controls the tact "I," we will contrast it with the public stimulus
that controls the tact "butterfly."

First, the person who experiences the butterfly (e.g., who is under
the stimulus control of the butterfly) can describe it in physical terms.

For example, the person might say, "It is about two inches wide, yellow and black, and has wings." These attributes are the characteristics of the public stimulus. The experience of "I," however, defies description in physical terms. A locus has no physical characteristics other than its relation to where the private activity of seeing takes place. Thus, the person might describe the physical characteristic of the *Sd* controlling "I" as lacking physical characteristics, such as "It is not my body." The locus remains constant even if the person grows from a child into an adult, changes jobs, or loses weight. The stimulus controlling "I," and therefore the experience of "I," remains constant even though the person's physical features and location may change. This characteristic is similar to the "featurelessness" of Deikman's description of the self.

Second, the butterfly has a specific location—over there, for example. The "I" is described as being within, the usual location of private stimuli, which is similar to Deikman's "central something."

Third, the butterfly's location can change from over there to over here. Given that the stimulus controlling "I" is always located where the private stimulation of seeing, wanting, feeling, and the like are, the "I" is experienced as always being in the same place. The butterfly can disappear whereas the "I" does not. Further, the butterfly changes over time—it ages and dies. Since the "I" is controlled by perspective which never changes, it is described as timeless. These characteristics resemble Deikman's definition of the self as "abiding" and "unchanging" and Erikson's notions of "selfsameness" and "continuity."

As stated previously, the self as an originator of action also appears in Masterson's and Deikman's descriptions of self. Our explanation of this aspect of the self experience involves learning that occurs after the emergence of "I" as a unit. This aspect of the self experience reflects perhaps a modern manifestation of primitive animism. *Animism* is a theory of the causes of behavior. Its fundamental assumption is that the source of every action can be attributed to the will of an actor. The animist explains actions by identifying the actor that is assumed to be present. Thus, to the animist, the activity of seeing must be attributed to an entity which originates it. Animistic theory seems to permeate the culture and people learn to attribute almost all actions to an instigating entity. The body could be one such entity which does the seeing, but this brings up the question of who makes the body act and the mind-body dilemma. The "I" that we have described is not experienced as one's body. Thus, to the animist that dwells in us all, an acceptable source of action would be the "I." From our perspective, of course, this does not make much sense. It is the same as saying "the originator of action is a locus."

Awareness also appears in definitions of the self. Deikman even said that the self *was* awareness. Translating into behavioral terms what we think Deikman was saying, awareness is the observation of our own behavior such that we can describe it. This is also described as *self-knowledge*. Thus, we would say that someone who says, "I see a butterfly," as opposed to, "That's a butterfly," has awareness. Other examples are "I drink," "I run," and "I say," which are tacts of one's own public behavior, and "I hear," "I want," and "I think," which are tacts of private behavior. A behavioral account of "higher levels of consciousness" (awareness) would involve iterations of the tacting of a tact of the private behaviors. For example, "I see myself seeing the butterfly," and "I see myself seeing myself see the butterfly."

How can this type of tacting lead to the experience described by Deikman that "I" is awareness? In our view, awareness is an activity and not a thing. On the other hand, the "I," or more precisely, the *Sd*s controlling "I," are a thing and not a behavior. Saying the self is awareness is like saying that a behavior is a thing or vice versa. In our everyday experience, however, things are equated with behavior when the two are closely associated. Since the behavior of being aware (i.e., tacting your own behavior) is very closely associated with the functional unit "I," the two are equated erroneously. Woodworth (cited in Catania, 1984) elaborated on the misleading nature of equating verbs with nouns:

> Instead of "memory" we should say "remembering;" instead of "thought" we should say "thinking" . . . But, like other learned branches, psychology is prone to transform its verbs into nouns. Then what happens? We forget that our nouns are merely substitutes for verbs, and go hunting for the things denoted by the nouns; but there are no such things, there are only the activities that we started with . . . remembering. (p. 303)

In summary, the particular stimuli that control the "I" response and the "I" feeling depend on the specific acquisition experiences as illustrated by our account of the emergence of the "I" response unit. Although normal development leads to a large degree of control of the "I" response by private stimuli, we propose that maladaptive development involves the opposite—a small degree of control of "I" by private stimuli.

MALADAPTIVE DEVELOPMENT OF THE SELF EXPERIENCE

We propose a continuum of severity of problems of the self based on the degree of private control of the "I" functional unit. One end of the continuum represents mild problems of the self that develop from insufficient private control over a small number of "I X" responses. Since "I" as a unit emerges from a large number of various "I X" units, the comparatively small number that are not privately controlled would have a negligible effect on the experience of self; that is, the self would be experienced as relatively unchanging, centrally located, and continuous. The larger the range of "I X" responses that the parents fail to bring under private control, however, the more problems one will experience with the self. Severe problems of the self are at the other end of the continuum that corresponds to a lack of private control over numerous "I X" units.

Problems of the self described in the psychoanalytic literature will be explored within our behavioral model. We have placed these self problems under the categories of "less severe" and "severe" to indicate roughly their position on the continuum of degree of private control over "I X" responses. These problems, however, are not mutually exclusive, and people with severe self disturbances are likely to experience the problems described under the "less severe" category in a more extreme way.

Less Severe Disturbances of the Self

People with mild to moderate self disturbances have a substantial number of "I X" responses evoked by private stimuli, but also have a significant number of such responses under partial or total public control. Thus, their sense of self can be greatly affected by the presence of other people and their opinions, moods, and desires. It is important to note that we are not talking about people who are unassertive or who know what they feel or want but have difficulty expressing it to others. Rather, we are describing a situation in which what a person feels or wants in the first place is under the control of others. In each of the problems described below, the degree of difficulty experienced by an individual will vary with the degree of private control over "I X" responses.

The Unstable or Insecure Self

If not enough "I Xs" are under private control, then the emergence of "I" as a functional unit is affected. As pointed out, in normal development the emerging "I" comes under the stimulus control of the locus where the activities such as seeing, wanting, feeling, thinking occurs. If these activities are partially under public control, then the experience of self will also be partially under public control. Since the public stimuli, such as parent behavior, can vary from time to time, the self experience will also vary depending on the degree to which it is publicly controlled. Thus, a somewhat insecure self will be experienced because it varies with who is present. In actuality, the publicly controlled self will vary more in close relationships. As we have described public control over "I X," it was a very important person—the parent—who became an *Sd*. In adult life, the self will correspondingly vary primarily with significant others. It is for this reason that intimate relationships may be a source of great conflict. For the individual with an unstable self, the avoidance of intimacy removes the source of the instability. The female client who feels okay about herself when she is alone but laments that she "loses herself" whenever she gets in a relationship is describing this phenomenon. Two subsets of this problem, difficulty in knowing what one wants and feels and extreme sensitivity to others, are described below.

1. *Difficulty in knowing what one wants and feels.* A parent who conditionally teaches his child to "I X," that is, only when the parent wants the child to do so, could be a behavioral description of the psychodynamic proposition that pathological development involves parents who have difficulty in separating their child's needs (reinforcers) from their own. The result of such experiences would be someone who has difficulty producing the "I want X" response in the absence of conspicuous public stimuli, such as the person asking that question also indicating what "should" be wanted. In this case, the problem of the self would mainly be experienced as "not knowing if what I want is really what *I* want or if it's just what *others* expect me to want."

As an example of how a person can punish or fail to reinforce a circumscribed set of "I want" responses, suppose a mother is with her toddler in a shopping mall and sees a cotton-candy machine. The mother is the one who wants the cotton candy, but instead of simply buying some, she prompts her child by saying, "Baby wants cotton candy." On the other hand, if baby says, "baby cot' candy," and the parent isn't in the mood, she may say, "No, baby doesn't want candy now." In addition to cotton candy, if this mother acts similarly with all sweets or treats, that is, she (1) prompts the child to say "I want ice cream" when she is really the one who wants the ice cream, and (2) she punishes the response otherwise (e.g., "you do not want ice cream, you just had some)," then for this child, "wanting treats" will not come under exclusive private control. The amount of private control will depend on how sensitive the mother is to her child's wanting treats.

At best, a conditional discrimination will be made in which the child will want treats only when two stimuli are present: (1) the private stimulus of wanting and (2) the public stimulus of her mother also wanting. When either is absent, the child will not want treats. At worst, her wanting treats will depend only on the particular wants of the mother at a particular time. When this child becomes an adult, a manifestation of her minor self problem is likely to occur as in this scenario: She is eating out with friends, and the waiter asks if she would like dessert. The adult looks puzzled, then turns to her friends and asks, "Do you want dessert?" and wants it only if they do.

A more problematic situation occurs when a wider spectrum of "I X" responses are not adequately brought under private control. In this case, the parent punishes or does not reinforce a range of responses that are normally controlled by stimuli accessible only to the child, such as "I want a pickle," "I have a tummy ache," "I feel like nobody loves me," "My dream was really scary," and "I want more." At worst, a severe self problem will develop in which the child will "want" or "feel" only when the parent or others indicate that it is all right to do so, and will have a hard time being in touch with his or her desires or feelings when alone. At best, a conditional "wanting" or "feeling" will occur that is under private control. In other words, when the child is alone, private stimuli will control the response, but when the parent is present, the child will avoid punishment and maximize reward by attending to the parent's reaction in order to come up with an acceptable response. Keep in mind that we are not referring to a child's suppressing a verbal report of feelings or needs. Rather, we are discussing the developmental antecedents of being aware of one's feelings and needs (reinforcers) and how one comes to notice and define one's feelings and needs in the first place.

In terms of reinforcement for the various types of verbal behavior, both the range and the consistency of responses would vary much more in the natural environment than in the simple explanatory examples we have provided. In general, as discussed in the chapter on emotions, we would expect greater inconsistency and undue reliance on public stimuli during the development of "I feel X," where X is an emotional reaction, hunger, or pain since these reactions are mainly private and their public aspects are subtle. In other words, even in adults with no or minimal self problems, their seemingly internal states can be greatly affected by external stimuli (e.g., feeling happy when in a jubilant crowd, not feeling hunger or a headache when intently working overtime to meet a deadline).

In general, the fewer the "I X" responses a person has under private control, the greater the confusion or difficulty he or she would experience in answering questions having to do with personal preferences, desires, and values when another person is present who is difficult to "read."

Such questions may include: "What do you like?" "What do you want?" "What do you believe?" and "What are your goals?"

2. *Extreme sensitivity to the opinions of others.* Extreme sensitivity to the opinions, beliefs, desires, and moods of others is another way of saying that a person's "I Xs" which should be under private control, are actually under public controlled. If a person's sense of self is shaky, any perceived or actual criticism may be experienced as devastating because it means any criticized "I Xs" were wrong or bad and the critic's "I Xs" must be adopted. It also involves a shift from whatever weak private control was present to control by the other. In some cases, criticism from a parent meant a major change in the parent's mood and thus became a discriminative stimulus for marked changes in the thinking, feeling, and seeing associated with "I X."

Life is unpredictable, chaotic, subject to the whims of others and is thus aversive under these conditions. An example of this sensitivity occurred during a therapy session with Irene and the first author. I meant to mildly chastise her by saying in a light and cheerful way, "Oh, come on Irene, you can do better than that" when she was less articulate than usual in answering a question. Although not apparent at the time, Irene later revealed she was devastated by my comment, withdrew into herself, and wanted to terminate therapy. If one's self mainly rests outside, that is control over the "I X" and "I" responses are publicly controlled, the overwhelming and all-encompassing nature of Irene's reaction makes sense.

A similar experience occurred with the second author and a client named Shelly who had been in therapy for a number of years. We were going through a "stuck" period, and I requested that Shelly should be more active in her therapy:

T: I'd like you to think about therapy goals between now and the next session so that we can talk about it then.

C: [*Looking agitated*] I don't know what you mean.

T: I don't have a clear enough sense of where you want to go, and I'd like you to take a more active role in that. Sometimes I feel like I have to work too hard to draw you out when you don't talk.

C: (*Tears stream down her face; she gets out of her chair and tries to leave the office*) I can't take this. I'm getting outa here.

T: No, Shelly, you are *not* going anywhere. Sit down and let's talk this out.

C: [*Sobbing and having a hard time getting her words out*] I didn't think anything was wrong. I thought I was doing a lot better with talking. I can't do what you want.

T: I am just trying to talk about ways to make your therapy better, and you're acting like I'm about to kick you out.

C: That's what it feels like, and I'm gonna leave you before you leave me.

T: I'm very committed to working with you, Shelly. Our relationship is not at all in jeopardy. That isn't the issue at all. I would like to be able to ask you to talk more or take more initiative without you threatening to quit therapy.

Because Shelly had a history of abandonment by significant others and suffered from an unstable sense of self, she reacted in an extreme way to my criticism of her. She felt as if her world had fallen apart because I did not perceive things the way she did. Because of my criticism, Shelly was confused about her "I Xs" and the only option was to adopt mine. Thus, therapy and I became unpredictable and threatening. In future sessions, I prompted and reinforced her for having different perceptions from me of how much she talked. As part of this process I encouraged her (1) to avoid tacting our differences as a matter of her being wrong and me being right and (2) to adopt the rule that my asking her to try to behave differently did not mean that I was going to abandon her if she did not or could not do what I asked (see Chapter 5 on cognitions and beliefs).

An analogy to Irene and Shelly's reactions using more concrete public stimuli would be: Person A says, "I see a mango," and person B says, "No, you don't, stupid, that's obviously an orange." If person A trusted her own perceptions, she would shrug off person B's comment as nuts, or would argue that B was the stupid one. But if person A did not trust her own perceptions (i.e., if her "I X" responses were not under solid private control) she would become upset and disoriented because her sense of the world was judged to be wrong.

Difficulty in Accessing the True Self, Spontaneity, and Creativity

When behavior has developed under the control of aversive stimuli, the source of the control is experienced as coming from outside and the person does not feel free (Skinner, 1971). *Aversive stimuli* refer to punishment, withdrawal of positive reinforcement, and threats of harm and deprivation. Thus, a child who grows up trying to please his parents because they will withdraw love if he does not, will feel as if he is being controlled by others. As discussed earlier, the use of aversive stimuli is almost always an instance of arbitrary reinforcement, and a child who grows up under the control of arbitrary reinforcement will also feel controlled and manipulated.

As used in our culture, a spontaneous act is one that is experienced as springing from within. Thus, the absence of spontaneous acts would correspond to a history dominated by aversive control. The unstable "I" could also play a role here. Just as it is possible for the "wants" of "I want" to be experienced as originating from the outside, so could the idea of "I have an idea," or the thoughts of "I think." If this type of public control is present, it would interfere with the experience of spontaneous action. Similarly, the sensitivity to criticism that characterizes the unstable "I" could limit spontaneity and creativity. Spontaneous and creative actions are members of a larger response class that contains weird, unusual, gross, obscene and other responses which are usually rejected by others. Thus, an increased sensitivity to criticism would result in a weakening of the whole response class including spontaneous and creative acts.

Narcissistic Personality Disorder

According to Kohut (1971, 1977), a person with narcissistic personality disorder experiences other people as undifferentiated from the individual who serves the needs of the self; that is, the narcissistic person fantasizes a control over others similar to the control an adult has over his or her own body. They are unable to rely on their own inner resources and therefore have created intense attachments to others.

There is a behavioral equivalent of narcissistic personality disorder that corresponds to Kohut's description. We hypothesize that narcissistic individuals grew up under typical conditions for unstable self-development (e.g., did not get consistent love or attention to emotional needs, were not consistently respected for their own experiences and views), but also were reinforced in limited or superficial ways for being charming, demanding, beautiful (usually in females) or powerful (usually in males). A person with such a background (1) would lack private control over "I," and thus would have difficulty differentiating someone else's needs from his or her own; (2) would have undue reliance on external reinforcers (e.g., others' praise and admiration, gifts) for a sense of self; and (3) would know how to control and manipulate others (e.g., through charm or power) to make relationships more tolerable.

An interesting hypothesis was proposed by Miller (1983) about the childhood histories of psychotherapists. She posited that the sensitivity to the needs of others and a desire to help those in distress, which are the qualities of a good psychotherapist, are originally shaped and reinforced by a narcissistic mother (the terms *shaping* and *reinforcement* are ours and are not used in Miller's writings). Obviously, in the case of a child who grows up to become a psychotherapist, the degree of narcissism would be limited as would be the disturbance of the self.

Severe Disturbances of the Self

A large number of "I X" responses under public control underlie severe self problems. This situation is produced by parents who are very inconsistent in their own reactions to conspicuous public stimuli (e.g., a schizophrenic or borderline parent). With such unstable parents, the "I see" response, for example, would be only reinforced when the following Sds were present: (1) the stimulus consisting of the child's public orienting to a public object, (2) the stimulus of the parent's publicly orienting, and (3) the stimulus of the parent not appearing to be preoccupied, distracted, or having a psychotic episode. Under these learning conditions, very little of the private activity of seeing would come to control the "I see" response. Instead, the child's seeing mainly would be controlled by the parent's mood and public orienting. Under these extreme circumstances, when the parent is present, the child would see a fish only if there were conspicuous public stimuli consisting of both a fish and indications the parent sees the fish.

The "I" that emerges under these conditions would be dependent on the cues provided by the parent. As a result, when the parent is present, what is seen, felt, wanted, liked, disliked, and so forth would be dependent on cues from that parent. For example, one set of cues may be that the parent appears to be in a good mood, is outwardly directed, and is paying attention to what is going on (e.g., the public stimuli), and gives indications that the child's needs will be attended to. Then, based on the child's past experiences of "father in a good mood," an extensive repertoire of "I X" responses, such as "I'm hungry" and "I just saw a birdie," will appear and be reinforced. The "I" that emerges under these conditions will be under public control; that is, the sense or experience of "I" is dependent on the cues given by the parent. When the parent is in a different state, however, withdrawn, inattentive, or even hallucinating, a different "I X" repertoire is called for and a different publicly controlled "I" experience would emerge (e.g., one that had no needs or feelings, or that is super-sensitive to the parents' needs). The diagnostic categories of borderline personality disorder and multiple personality disorder, discussed below, represent severe disorders of the self.

Borderline Personality Disorder

The statement, "I feel empty," which is characteristic of clients who are diagnosed as having borderline personality disorder, could be an effect of the relative absence of private Sds which control "I." Since wanting, feeling, thinking, and the like are mainly not under private control in the extreme pathological case, the locus is primarily outside and dependent on the parent's behavior. The "outside" location of the stimuli evoking "I" would be experienced as depersonalization, and when these external stimuli are absent, one would experience the absence or loss of self. Since *emptiness* refers to something that was contained within and is now gone, the presence and absence of the stimuli controlling the experience of self would be tacted as "emptiness."

According to Linehan (1987), an invalidating parental environment leads to the development of borderline personality disorder. Such parents are likely to (1) invalidate the child's reports of current emotional experiences, especially negative ones (i.e., not take them seriously, disbelieve the reports, respond as if the child is not feeling what he or she communicates); (2) oversimplify the ease of controlling one's emotional experiences, thinking, and action, and thus invalidate the child's experiences of difficulty and need for help; and (3) excessively criticize or respond punitively when the child expresses preferences, values, and beliefs that do not reflect those of the parents.

The behavioral view of Linehan's account is that invalidation is the lack of positive reinforcement for the private control of the child's responses. As she describes it (but in our words), this interferes with private control over a broad range of "I X" responses, such as "I want," "I feel," "I need," and "I believe." As pointed out, these contingencies will not only directly affect the experience of "I want," "I feel," "I need," and "I believe," but will also affect the "I" experience that emerges from these.

To illustrate this model, we turn to Angela, a client who described what it was like going grocery shopping with her mother. She recalled that most of the time her mother was cruel and rejecting. She remembered sitting in the shopping cart and feeling her usual detachment and bewilderment. On one of those infrequent occasions in which her mother was kinder and more nurturing, however, Angela was asked if she wanted a treat. Her detachment disappeared, and she had a sudden awareness of all the goodies that she wanted and she excitedly asked for one. Thus, controlled by the public stimulation of her mother's behavior, Angela's "seeing," "wanting," and sense of self appeared.

What was observed in Angela's case were the effects of publicly controlled "I Xs" on the discontinuous and unstable sense of self. The case is also an example of Angela's extreme sensitivity to the moods of others. Specifically, a relatively small change in her mother's behavior served as a discriminative stimulus for marked changes in the thinking, feeling, and seeing associated with "I X."

What is the "I" experience when no significant other is present? In the normal environment where "I" eventually comes under private control, the "I" experience would be similar in all situations. In the maladaptive environment, however, the absence of the parent would remove stimuli evoking "I" so that one either lost the sense of self, or developed a sense of self that was distinct from the self or the selves evoked by others. The explanation of how this "alone" self might develop is related to the more general case of how talking to oneself is reinforced and maintained—a topic discussed Chapter 5 on cognition. Based on the notions from Chapter 5, there are times when making certain "I X" statements to one's self would be of value (reinforced). For example, saying to oneself "I'm tired and need to rest" could be helpful in signaling when it is time to rest. In these cases, the reinforcement is more likely to be natural and thus consistent. The alone self that was developed under these conditions would be more consistent and unchanging although it might be less extensive then one developed on a broader base of "I X."

A description of how an absent self can fare when alone was provided by Tom, a client who often withdrew and retreated into himself. During these retreats, according to Tom, he could relax and be himself. A day could pass with little awareness of what was going on around him. Although he seemed to have little sense of self when alone, this self was experienced as stable, not subjected to the whims of others, and therefore was a positive experience for him. In contrast, he found it intrusive to disrupt the state in order to relate to his therapist or his wife. He remembered first doing these withdrawals during his chaotic childhood and continued to do it whenever possible.

Avoidance of those situations in which "I" is publicly controlled would follow if, as in a case like Tom's, one can only be "relaxed" when "I" is not being controlled by another. One form of this avoidance would be to avoid all others and become a hermit. A more practical form is to just avoid those relationships in which the other exerts control over "I." From our perspective, whenever the reactions of others are important sources of reinforcement, the others can control "I." Thus, meaningful, close, and significant relationships are avoided. As Angela described it, she lost her identity whenever she or the other person started to "care." "When this happens," she said, "it's time to split."

On the other hand, many people who have little private control over "I" find it almost intolerable to be alone. We hypothesize that in addition to the invalidating conditions that interfered with their development of "I," they were also subjected to extreme neglect in which basic needs were not met (e.g., as infants and toddlers, they were left hungry, thirsty, soiled, cold, and scared for long periods of time). For these people, extreme neglect occurred because the parent was absent and/or nonattentive. The absent self, on the other hand, was also evoked by the absent and/or nonattentive parent. Under these circumstances, the conditions that evoked an absent self are frightening. With such backgrounds, they would seek out constant companions, not only to escape the emptiness, but also to avoid the panic associated with previous neglect experiences.

It is not uncommon for individuals with little or no sense of self to crave both aloneness and companionship. One such client, Penny, would engage in a series of one-night stands to escape her inner void, but as soon as someone became a more steady part of her life, she would feel angry and suffocated and would drive him away. Her behavior made sense because she was subjected to an invalidating environment with both aversive control *and* abandonment/neglect experiences in her childhood.

Multiple Personality Disorder

Multiple personality disorder (MPD) is the diagnosis applied to an individual who acts as though he or she is more than one person. At various times, the MPD patient may speak, emote, remember, and experience the self in ways that normally are only seen in different individuals. Our impressions about the nature and treatment of MPD that are presented in this section are largely based on the comprehensive text by Putnam (1989).

Although relatively little is known about this complex and puzzling disorder, the etiological factor of childhood trauma is well accepted. One study, for example, found that 97% of all MPD patients reported experiencing severe trauma in childhood (National Institute of Mental Health, cited in Putnam). These traumas included sexual and/or physical abuse, extreme neglect, and witnessing violent death.

The prototypic MPD case involves the following: during severe abuse, the child experiences leaving the scene or depersonalization, something like an out-of-body experience in which the child perceives himself floating above his body or going to another place. Later, and often throughout life, the details of the abuse are forgotten; that is, there is amnesia of the abuse. In the argot of the MPD literature, the self that experiences leaving the scene and has amnesia is referred to as the *host*. Even though the host is gone, however, another aspect of the self is present and aware of the details of the abuse while it is happening. This aspect of the self is referred to as an *alter* (or *alters*, since usually more than one exists). Awareness by one alter of the others can also be circumscribed or absent.

The repertoires of behavior that define the host and alter(s) have many characteristics of separate persons. Whether they are considered to be separate depends on the definition of a person or individual. If the definition includes a single body, then the host and alter cannot be considered separate. If, however, a behavioral definition is used, it is then possible to consider the multiples as more or less separate persons. A person can be defined in terms of his or her characteristic way of acting, including style of talking, style of interpersonal relating, assertiveness, special skills (e.g., a printer, a physician), memories (remembering), as well as their reinforcers (interests, values, preferences, and the like). Additionally, an individual person's experience of the self includes continuity, an abiding awareness, and an originator of actions. In other words, one experiences oneself as the locus in which seeing, hearing, and remembering occur. This locus is differentiated from other people's locuses. From a behavioral viewpoint, the host and alters can thus be considered separate persons to the extent to which they have the behavioral characteristics of separate persons. The fact that it is at least possible for an alter to know the private experiences of the host, however, is a behavioral characteristic that is not found in separate persons.

The separate personlike nature of the host and alters is dramatically illustrated when an alter is violent and persecutory. Putnam reported that many serious suicide attempts (and presumably some suicides) are the result of homicidal behavior of an alter directed at the host and/or other alters. On the other hand, some alters have only a few characteristics of another person, and are referred to in the MPD literature as personality fragments. For example, the alter may be an infant with very limited repertoires. For clinicians who have not had direct experience with MPD, it is perhaps difficult to accept the notion that an alter (e.g., a person whose individuality is defined by his or her behavior) can be experienced by others (the therapist) as a separate person. Both authors have treated MPD clients and can corroborate the reports of other clinicians that the host and alters are frequently experienced as different individuals. This is consistent with the behavioral view that, in many ways, they are separate persons.

The possibility that MPD can be feigned must also be considered, and there have been documented cases of this phenomenon. It has also been suggested that MPD is an iatrogenic disorder; that is, therapists who are looking for the novelty and drama of MPD might inadvertently suggest and reinforce this behavior in their clients. Even if not directly suggested or encouraged, treating the alters as separate persons provides contingencies to maintain their separateness. Some support for the role of contingencies in MPD was demonstrated by Kohlenberg (1973), who showed that the various personalities of a patient appeared and disappeared when reinforced for doing so. Although malingering and iatrogenic contingencies must be considered, evidence suggests that most cases of MPD are not conjured up for the therapist's benefit. In particular, the diagnosis of the disorder and the discovery of alters often occur after 5 years or more of therapy. Since the adaptive value of MPD is closely tied to secrecy and deception, it is possible that many or even most cases are never diagnosed.

A behavioral account of MPD. We will explore the applicability of our behavioral conception of self to the various phenomena of MPD. These phenomena include the distinct repertoires of behavior and the experience of self that characterize MPD. An account of MPD should also show why this reaction to stress occurs only in childhood and point to possible individual differences that explain why the disorder does not develop in all severely traumatized children.

We assume that before the trauma, the child has already developed repertoires of behavior that predispose him or her to MPD. Then, at the time of the trauma, these repertoires are called into play and MPD develops.

First, the self at the time of trauma is not completely under private control. In a sense, the theory of self presented in this chapter is a theory of how we come to experience our self as an individual person in the first place. Before private stimuli come to control "I," some characteristics of an individual (e.g., a single personality) have not emerged. Specifically, the child has a relatively diminished experience of the self as (1) continuous, (2) an originator of actions, and (3) an abiding resting awareness that sees all. For these states to occur, the parent must consistently reinforce "I X" responses so that the locus gains control. Before this normal process is completed, a wide variety of self experiences are possible.

Since the developing child is more prone to changes in the experience of self, the norm is a fluctuating self. For example, when cuddling with her father, a little girl may be quiet, controlled, and subdued, but when playing with other children, she turns into an altogether different character. She may become loud, uncontrolled, and aggressive. Not only do these observable repertoires shift, but the child will also experience these selves as separate (to the extent that her "I" experience is under public control). We believe the activity of "being someone else" is facilitated by these normal childhood experiences of separate selves.

The activity of being someone else is often seen in children. They play games of pretend in which they are adults, doctors, witches, daddy, or mommy. They are exposed to the public stimuli of seeing their parents' actions, being read a description of characters in a story, or seeing cartoon personalities on TV. These characters are public stimuli that model how children could act, feel, and see. With a little prompting and encouragement, a child often adopts these roles. At any shopping center, toddlers can be seen wearing Batman capes and jumping off benches, swaggering around in cowboy boots, chaps, and hat, or making sputtering noises and swooping around like an airplane. The paraphernalia show that parents often prompt and reinforce this activity. Although adults can also engage in "being someone else," we are suggesting that the experience is different for children. Since the child has a more malleable self, the experience is more real in that a wider range of "I X" activities can also be affected. That is, the child might actually experience the feelings and visual images of being big, strong, and agile like Batman (the MPD client, incidentally, may actually see different persons when looking in a mirror, depending on which alter is present). In contrast, the adult actor is more in contact with a stable sense of self and visual experiences that remind her or him of being an ordinary person who is playing the role of someone else.

Other contingencies may also help to maintain being someone else. A boy may be directly encouraged by the parent to act like someone else when he is told, "Go out there and be a man." Being someone else also seems to be reinforced when playing with other children as in cops and robbers. Of relevance to the present topic, however, being someone else also may be reinforced because it reduces the aversiveness of punishment. For example, if a boy is sent to his room, and when there pretends to be Superman, this pretense can distract the child from the aversive conditions that brought him to be in the room. Keep in mind that the activity of pretending by a child whose "I" is still controlled by public stimuli can change the fundamental experience of what is seen and felt.

The malleability of self that conforms to the demands of public stimuli is also demonstrated by the increased susceptibility to suggestion found in children. Children, as a group, are significantly more hypnotizable than adults (Putnam, 1989, p. 52). We are viewing hypnotizability as the responsiveness to public control over what is seen and otherwise experienced (e.g., hypnotic suggestions in the form of "You feel your eyelids getting heavier and heavier." "You are getting warmer." "You see a star in a distant galaxy whizzing toward you, and it is getting bigger and brighter.") Again, as the child matures, there is relatively less control by public stimuli, the self is more stable, and hypnotizability declines.

In terms of the role of trauma, when a highly aversive event repeatedly occurs, the child is motivated to escape and avoid. Since running away or striking out at the abuser is ineffective, other avoidance or escape repertoires would emerge. Being someone else might be such a repertoire; that is, if the child is experienced in being someone else, it could be functional to do this at the time of trauma. This is particularly true if being someone else were already effective for reducing aversiveness (as in the example of the boy being sent to his room as punishment). In addition to reducing aversiveness through distraction, the particular someone else the child is pretending to be might also help avoid aversiveness by having limited awareness (such as an infant) or increased pain tolerance (such as Superman).

Being someone else during the trauma would be particularly adaptive if the host does not remember what happened (amnesia). As discussed in Chapter 4, remembering is a behavior that is subject to its consequences as is any operant behavior. Even without being someone else, traumatic events often are not remembered. Remembering is facilitated by contact with the stimuli related to the event being remembered. Not remembering is aided by the avoidance of those situations that remind. Being someone else who sees differently than the primary self in effect changes the stimuli that are seen and thus avoids contact with stimuli related to the event being remembered. This, in turn, facilitates the amnesia. Perhaps the primary function of being someone else during the trauma is that it facilitates amnesia in this way.

Becoming someone else during the trauma and then switching and not remembering has the effect of isolating the traumatic event. If the amnesia did not happen, then the effects of the trauma would be more intrusive in the daily life of the child, which is the case with adult posttraumatic stress disorder. Thus, the child would be fearful and would avoid the abuser and everything else connected with the trauma. This type of avoidance would not be adaptive because usually the abuser is the parent or caretaker. The child is therefore dependent on the abuser and must live in the environment where the abuse occurred. Instead, with isolation of the trauma, the child can even be loving or affectionate to the abuser most of the time and thus receive the attention necessary for survival.

Once isolation of the trauma occurs, the development of the self is fragmented. Rather than an increasing amount of private control of a single "I," there is more than one "I" that can be controlled by different private stimuli, and there can be more than one locus or perspective. In addition to the locus of the "I" for the host, there can be a different locus where the alter's seeing occurs. These multiple sources of control over "I" could be expected to influence the experience of the location of the self. This situation might also contribute to the frequent out-of-body experiences that are reported by MPD clients, which they often describe as like watching a movie or looking down at themselves from above. The separate experiences of the host and alters allow for independent development of almost any aspect of a person. Thus, each alter can have its own likes and dislikes, vocabulary, experience of self, visual experiences, and the like. Some of the alters are static in their development because of their limited contact with the world and remain the same age as when first formulated. Other alters are in more contact with the world and change or mature with experience.

MPD treatment issues. The way in which the therapist is supposed to relate to the alters is a major issue in treatment and leads to conflicting advice. On the one hand, Putnam (1989) emphasized that the alter personalities are not separate people and should always be treated as parts of the same individual. On the other hand, when Putnam gave the details of treatment, the opposite seems to be the case. For example, in detailing treatment procedures, Putnam encouraged the therapist to ask the alters what their names were, to enlist the aid of one alter in controlling another, to not play favorites, and to ask for everyone's attention when the therapist had an important announcement.

There is a good rationale, however, for each of the contradictory approaches to the alters. On the one hand, treatment is aimed at some kind of integration or unification. Treating the alters as separate persons undermines this goal. Yet, on the other hand, a necessary part of therapy involves accessing the secret alters, and they will remain secret unless treated like separate persons. Sizemore (1989), who is the "Eve" of the well-known *Three Faces of Eve*, described the importance of the clinician's accepting the alters as real: "With clinicians viewing the alters of MPD patients as parts or fragments or illusions but the patients viewing their alters as other people, basic communication was breaking down" (p. 267). Our behavioral conceptual model seems to offer a way out of this dilemma and also points to some general therapeutic directions.

In terms of behavior, the alters are more or less separate persons. Therefore, they should be treated in therapy in accordance with the type of person they are. An alter who describes herself as 6 years old would be treated differently than one who is a bristly adolescent. The goal in treatment is to bring the alters into more awareness of each other's experiences. Often this process is highly aversive and evokes avoidance; that is, it can be very anxiety provoking to the host to be told that she is a multiple much less than to be told the details of an alter's experience. Just as in family therapy, patience and caution are required in getting the alters to reveal their innermost thoughts and discuss them with others. This is particularly true in MPD since the reason the alters came into being was to hide information. Over the course of therapy, the therapist offers help to alters in much the same way that it would be offered to any other client. Attention to CRB is always important. Of course, the biggest CRB1 is the lack of awareness and distinctive repertoires that are characteristic of MPD. Other CRB1 are anger toward the therapist by an alter who is also angry at other alters and at other people in daily life. As the alters improve and increase their awareness of one another, the therapist can fade her or his role as a mediator. Gradually, the repertoires of the alters would become more alike and the client's behavior would become more like that of an individual person. Therapy is considered successful when such clients are effective in their daily lives, even if they do not necessarily experience the single self that most people experience. Sizemore (1989) described her posttherapy experience in the following manner: "Even terms like unification or integration seem to reinforce an unnatural view of self. Because even if the integrated MPD patient accepts these clinical terms on an intellectual basis, the patient still possesses what is best described as an unconscious conviction: Once I was many. Now I am one. But I am not the puzzle put together from their parts." (p. 267) Or, as suggested by Putnam, the posttherapy experience of MPD could be like that of an effective partnership or corporation. At the annual international conference on MPD and dissociative disorders held in Chicago, the second author was particularly moved by a therapist with MPD who spoke in a workshop about her healing experiences. She stated that she was now integrated, but that every day she meditated and visualized each of her alters, telling them, "I will never forget you, and I will never forsake you."

CLINICAL IMPLICATIONS

In broad terms, clients with extensive problems of the self start treatment with in-session behaviors of being wary, overly attentive, and concerned about the therapist's opinion of them, and do not confidently describe feelings, beliefs, wants, likes, and dislikes. All these behaviors are likely to be CRB1s, which indicate a lack of private control over internal stimuli. If treatment is successful, their within-session behaviors become confident and trusting, and include the CRB2s of freely describing thoughts, feelings, wants, and beliefs.

The description of client behaviors articulated in the foregoing paragraph could pass for the generic client problem and the generic psychotherapeutic endeavor. This observation combined with the burgeoning literature on the development and treatment of self problems probably reflect the prevalence of problems of the self. Since a primary source of the client's difficulties is the lack of private control, treatment by a therapist who is accepting, responsive, and who encourages "expression or release of feelings" could naturally provide the contingencies to strengthen private control. Such a generic therapeutic environment is the antidote to the invalidating parental environment that failed to reinforce control by private stimuli. In addition, our behavioral model leads to some specific suggestions (discussed below) that can enhance the more general psychotherapy.

Reinforce Talking in the Absence of Specific External Cues

For clients with self problems, much of their behavior is under the tight stimulus control of others. They appear vigilant and are focused intently on the therapist, watching for every nuance in facial expression and voice inflection. Although often not obvious at first, almost everything the clients say about themselves and what they think and feel may be heavily influenced by the discriminative control of the therapist. The therapy procedure we will describe is aimed at loosening this control by encouraging and reinforcing talking in the absence of specific external cues. In other words, treatment consists of strengthening the CRB2s of privately controlled "I X," which would also aid in the eventual emergence of private control over "I."

One way to help clients establish private control is to take the psychoanalytic stance of passivity, not to structure each moment of the session with questions. This will certainly enhance the chances of evoking CRB2—"I X" responses under private control. At least in the beginning stages of treatment, this kind of strategy is problematic in two ways. First, it could evoke a strong CRB1 of avoidance and accompanying overwhelming emotional responses that ultimately result in clients fleeing treatment. We have had numerous clients who complained bitterly about previous treatment failures because of their ex-therapists' passivity.

Second, this tactic is likely to preclude the therapist's reinforcing of CRB2, should it occur. For example, the client might say, "I can't stand this." This type of statement is an "I X" response that should be reinforced by the therapist who should take it seriously, whereas maintaining passivity probably would not be reinforcing. A more or less passive therapist, however, might be just what the doctor ordered in a later stage of therapy after clients have made some progress in gaining a self or a privately controlled repertoire of "I X" responses. At the other extreme, a highly active therapist who avoids evoking any client anxiety will make the client feel and perform all right during the session, but will preclude the likelihood of CRB2's occurring. An ideal therapy would be highly structured in the beginning and gradually become unstructured as it progresses.

To illustrate the points just made, let us turn to a male client named Terry. During the initial months of therapy with the first author, Terry focused mainly on his medical treatment and the medications he was using to control a psychosomatic symptom. When I posed more general questions about mood or any emotional state, Terry became stymied and anxious. At first, I would help by suggesting a specific answer based on specific public stimuli. For example, when a new, severe medical symptom appeared that was similar to one that resulted in a relative's death, I suggested that Terry was feeling fear; that is, I provided the public stimulus by saying "fear." This is quite similar to what parents do when they impart to their children the tacts for emotions. Early in the course of treatment, I made many similar suggestions of specific feelings for specific situations. Gradually, over the next few months, the specificity was reduced. Rather than continue to give a specific feeling, I would give him a list to choose from (e.g., pain, fear, anger, disappointment, irritation, or frustration). In other words, I was still prompting a response based on public stimuli, but the specificity of the stimuli was broadened. Terry was assured that he would not be punished for answering since he was given an "approved" answer in the first case and a "list" of approved answers in the second. The general idea was that structure was gradually reduced to allow more of the private stimuli to gain control.

Match Therapeutic Tasks to the Level of Private Control in the Client's Repertoire

In order to vary the amount of public control over client behavior, we use a variant of free association as a technique. Just as the general strategy of a therapist can vary from passive to highly structured, the free association task can be presented with more or less structure. When used in FAP, the primary purpose of free association is not to uncover hidden meanings or to make use of the content although the content is sometimes relevant. Instead, it is the behavior of free associating that is of interest. In its most unstructured form, the free association instructions are: "Tell me everything which enters your mind—all thoughts, feelings, and images. It's important not to censor anything. Report whatever comes up, even if you think it's unimportant nonsensical, trivial, embarrassing, or whatever." The client is asked to continue to do this without feedback from the therapist and may even be asked to sit so that the therapist is out of view.

Our view of this task is that it requires talking to another person (the therapist) with a minimum of external cues from the listener. Under these conditions it is possible for the client to say "I feel X" or "I see this image" under conditions that favor control by private stimuli. As illustrated in the case given below, clients with extensive self problems will become very anxious and be unable to perform this task because of the lack of public stimulation. They may actually experience a "loss of self" in the absence of therapist cues. A similar phenomenon occurs when behavior therapists use relaxation or meditation techniques and find that their clients become highly anxious when the task is too unstructured. So, when using free association during FAP, variations in the classical unstructured format are often employed. A series of free-association type tasks are used that involve a gradually increasing degree of private control. The initial tasks are sentence completion and word association. Then, tasks involving mental imagery and self-observation of private responses are introduced.

A more structured variant of free association is the "movie theater in your mind" task. Clients are asked to close their eyes and to imagine they are sitting in a movie theater. First they are instructed to see a blank screen in their minds' eye. Then, when the movie starts, the first scene is stipulated to be of the client and the therapist sitting in the office at that very moment. Next, the movie is described running backward with the client walking backward out of the office and back into his car. The movie is then said to run faster and faster, turning into a blur. The client is asked to view the blur and have it suddenly stop and to describe the scene. It would be important, of course, to reinforce any "I X" responses because they are likely to be under at least a modicum of private control. There are a wide variety of such imagery tasks used in gestalt therapy, psychosynthesis, and hypnotherapy that can be adapted for FAP.

Another adaptation of free association involves the use of a computer and word processor. The client is asked to type everything that crosses her or his mind and not to censor anything. An advantage of this method is that it lends itself to shaping the process. At first, the client is given the option of erasing any or all the material before the therapist reviews it. In order to reinforce talking (typing) in the absence of public stimuli, the therapist uncritically reviews the word processing file during the session. Over time, the client is encouraged to erase as little as possible.

We will illustrate the principle of matching therapeutic tasks with the level of client private control with the case of Fred, a 34-year-old physicist. He was often overwhelmed with anxiety in significant personal and work relationships when he felt criticized or rejected. When criticized, or when afraid he would be criticized, he would disappear, dissociate, and shirk his responsibilities. Obviously, such behavior resulted in his being in trouble at work, yet he would be unaware that he had caused any problems. In addition, Fred generally was withdrawn and tried to avoid human interaction. He had difficulty in knowing how he felt; that is, he lacked "I feel X" responses which were under private control. Fred had been termed "alexythymic" (unable to express feelings) by a previous therapist. Not surprisingly, Fred remembered both his mother and father to be cold, demanding, explosive, disapproving, and unaffectionate parents.

In a session with the first author, Fred was given a time-limited version of free association.

T: What we'll do is I'll just ask you to close your eyes and then all I want you to do is report to me what kind of images or feelings, or thoughts, or memories occur. So if you're getting a blurry something, just say "I'm seeing a blurry whatever." So you kind of give me a running dialogue of whatever is going on, including if nothing is going on.
(The client is being prompted to give "I X" responses, and is being reassured that any response is okay.)

C: Okay. (A long, long pause.) Terrible (half laughter).
(Fred doesn't do as requested.)

T: What's going on?

C: I, I just can't (A long pause.) I mean, it's, I mean, I can't, I can't focus, it's really embarrassing, you know, you ought to be able to do it.

T: What was your experience, when you closed your eyes, what happened?

C: I mean, it's just, it's just like nothing, you know, I mean . . .
(He is describing a private event—nothing happened.)

T: A total, a total blank?

    (This was probably not the best response to reinforce privately controlled behavior.)

C: Yeah.

T: Well, that's okay, that's fine. I'd like you to tell me there is nothing. You also said it was terrible, so at some point you must also have been feeling like this was terrible, is that right?

    (An attempt to remedy the possible punishment in the previous response by saying it's okay to report having a blank mind. Also a prompt of "I feel terrible" based on the presence of the public stimulus—his comment "terrible.")

C: Yeah.

T: So, what you would do is say something like, "I'm not seeing anything," that would be fine, and "I'm feeling terrible, or I'm feeling this is terrible because I should be able to see something." See, what I'm asking you to report is everything that is going on, imagery or no imagery, how you're feeling and what you're saying to yourself about this.

    (Prompting of "I X.")

C: I think what's happening there is, uh, I have to be able to back off a little bit, I mean, and I even try to do that and I'm having some trouble.

    (Fred is indicating how difficult the task is. I understood the backing off comment to be a type of self-awareness response. But I also took it as a disguised mand for me to back off.)

T: You're having trouble backing off to tell me about it?

C: Right. Yeah, just [pause], you know, being an observer in this situation.

T: So, when your eyes are closed it's kind of like you're having this experience, and you can't pull back from that, is that what you're saying? You can't watch yourself having this experience?

C: Right.

T: Okay, are you willing to do this? Are you willing to keep your eyes closed for 5 minutes, and I won't say anything to you. What you will do is experience what you are experiencing and then try to tell me what you are experiencing. So, you may be silent for 5 minutes in the sense that you may never be able to pull back. Maybe 5 minutes is too long; I'd say 2 minutes. Let's do it 2 minutes. So do you want to have a run on it for 2 minutes?

    (Restructuring the task. An advantage to viewing the task as instructions to evoke privately controlled responses is that the therapist can modify it on the spot in any way that would seem to help toward the goal.)

C: Okay, I think [pauses], I think part of the problem I have with that intuitively is that I don't want to be out of contact with you.

    (This comment reveals how important it is to Fred to have feedback from another in order to do a task which is intended to be under private control.

Note also that it is a CRB3, an important and rare description of the variables controlling Fred's avoidance and anxiety.)

T: When you are out of contact, then you get anxious.

C: Yeah, I think it would just simply get worse. The longer it went on.

T: Makes sense. Makes sense to me. Does it to you?

(It makes sense to me as a radical behaviorist who has a theory about how an invalidating parent affects control over public and private stimulation.)

C: Not too much.

(About 5 minutes of conversation.)

C: What is this sort of telling you? It makes sense to you but I'm not sure it makes sense to me.

T: Well, it has to do with the fact that I am a significant person for you. And I think it shows a basic fear that you have in relationships with significant people. I think you need to see the other person's reactions because if you have to rely on just your own sense, you'll read it wrong and you'll be in big trouble.

(I am attempting a behavioral interpretation that describes the troublesome discriminative stimuli [Sds] involving significant others, the history of reinforcement involving punishment for private control, and the avoidance of punishment for being under public control.)

C: Yeah, I think that.

T: I think that's the way to describe it in terms of making sense. But, knowing that, I don't think is going to help you, I think it's very unconscious. I mean, I think you just feel this way, and so I say it makes sense in that it reflects your history.

(Here I am putting interpretation and "knowledge" in their place as aiding in rule-governed behavior and acknowledging the contingency-shaped nature of the problem.)

C: Yeah it does.

T: But I would see this as being pretty important to you to try and overcome that (needing to be in contact).

C: Yeah. [*pauses*] I'm trying to figure out some way of getting around that (needing to be in contact). You know, I think probably I'm more aware of barriers. I'm just becoming more and more aware of it. I think this is a pretty high barrier, well, my mind says you've got to engineer your way around that or engineer a solution.

(Fred is describing his increased awareness of the private experience of the barrier. The barrier gives an indication of the intensity of feelings generated by the lack of public stimuli.)

T: Yeah, that was kind of my thinking, too.

C: Well, if we did it in chunks, maybe increasing time, and then if I explained if I remember, and don't edit afterward . . .

(Here is a CRB2 of suggesting a solution to a barrier rather than dissociating.)

T: Right. So should we try a 15-second chunk?

C: Sure.

T: Okay. Start. (A 15-second pause.) Time's up.

C: [*mumble*] The barrier definitely lasts, I think.

T: What was going on while your eyes were closed?

C: I really didn't have, I mean, again, I just, just this white I mean, just this blur, but it's sort of like there's something swirling there that, uh, maybe was my level of anxiety was not as high.

(This is an "I X" report, Fred's most elaborated report of the imagery experience to this point.)

(A few minutes later.)

T: So, this process that we went through, just in the last few minutes was not anything you're used to. The process was this, I had an expectation that was too much for you. You got very anxious about it, we talked about it, and came up with a different approach which was tailored to fit more where you are at. And you were able to do better at the imagery task. This process is not anything like what happened between you and your father. Now this is also related to something you run into at work. They ask you to do something, if you can't do it you just freeze up.

(Following Rule 5, I make an interpretation based on events that just occurred. The situation, history, behavior, and consequences are given and related to daily life.)

C: That's true. I guess, it feels like I made a little progress there for me.

T: Right. I think so, too.

In summary, four adjustments should be made to imagery or free association tasks borrowed from other therapies. First, they should be presented to the client as a task whose value is derived from the process (e.g., imagining and describing in the presence of the therapist). Ideally, clients should be told, in everyday terms, that what is important about the task is that it is likely to evoke CRB2s under private control. Second, the task should be selected or modified to vary in the degree of private control required to match the level of the client's repertoire. For example, the "movie theater" task, could start with no image present on the screen or could be time-limited. Third, the client should be reinforced for making "I X" statements. Prompting of "I X" statements, as illustrated in Fred's case, should also be used if needed. Fourth, the therapist should keep in mind that CRBs other than those related to self problems could be evoked and provide certain therapeutic opportunities. For example, in Terry's case, the imagery task not only evoked CRB related to the self, but also to the problems he had at work when coping with tasks that were too difficult.

Reinforce as Many Client "I X" Statements as Possible

It is extremely important to treat with respect all of the client's ideas, intuitions, theories, and beliefs that differ from yours. What we mean by respect is that the client's behavior should be strengthened by your reaction even though you may indicate you feel differently. Ideally, the therapist's reaction should be positively reinforcing even if it also reflects a different opinion than the client's. Special significance is given to those client "I X" statements that differ from yours because it is precisely these behaviors that are most likely to be under private control. The idea is to reinforce as many "I Xs" as possible.

As we have stated previously, if the client's self problem is related to a lack of private control over "I want," it is critical to reinforce, if at all possible, such a response if it occurs. One important clue that a client's "I want" is under private control (as opposed to public control—e.g., the therapist's control) is the therapist's inclination to reject the request.

For example, a client whose self problem was that she did not know what she wanted and could not say what she wanted, asked the first author to try hypnosis to find out what she wanted. My first reaction was to turn her down and give the reasons why I did not use hypnosis. Using my inclination to reject her request as a cue that signaled the possibility that her "want" was under private control, my next reaction was to privately recognize that her request was a CRB2. Seeing that this was something that *she* truly wanted, I then changed my mind and agreed to hypnotize her.

Another example can be seen in the case of a female client who lost her identity when she was in an intense relationship with a man. She also developed an intense relationship with the first author and told me about her paranormal experiences. Even though I personally did not believe in them, I recognized her behavior as CRB2 and was quite genuinely thrilled with her telling me about her beliefs.

For clients who do not know how they feel, it may be important in the earliest stages of treatment for the therapist to help them figure out how they feel. By doing so, the therapist provides an experience similar to that which occurs in Stage I. By responding to public stimuli in much the same way a parent does when teaching the child to tact feelings, the therapist assists in building in tacts of feelings. The external cues used by the therapist could be the physical appearance of the client (e.g., the client might appear quite tense, tired, anxious, or depressed). The therapist then says, "You look tired " or "depressed" or whatever the case might be.

Another external cue is the nature of the therapeutic interaction that has just occurred. For example, a therapist who persisted in asking the client to talk about an unpleasant event even though the client did not want to might suggest that the client feels "pushed around," irritated, or resentful because of the persistence. The therapist would then encourage the client to say, "I feel X." The danger in using this procedure is that the therapist might persist in this approach for too long, rely too much on public stimuli, and thus preclude or interfere with the client's gaining private stimulus control. Although our discussion has focused on clients who do not know how they feel, similar procedures can be used in the early stages of therapy for clients who do not know what they want, or believe, or know.

A delicate juncture is broached when a client whose self problems include a paucity of "I feel" responses and who says, "I feel you don't care about me." Such a client comment is not unusual and should be treated as an instance of CRB2 (assuming it is not a disguised mand for reassurance). It is important for the therapist to take the comment seriously and not to punish a CRB2 by terming such a reaction as *transference* or making an interpretation that the client's response is not based on anything that happened in the session, but that comes instead from childhood. Rather, the most reinforcing response would be to validate why the client may feel that way. Therefore, it is incumbent on the therapist to carefully review past events in the therapy and to look within to find the events that might support the client's observation.

For example, the therapist may have been distracted or preoccupied during the session or may even have been irritated by the client. Needless to say, this validation of the client's tact does not preclude the importance of the therapist's emphasizing his of her caring of the client in general.

An even more difficult situation is encountered when a client comes up with "I X" statements that are counterproductive, self-maligning, suicidal, or homicidal. Our suggestions for dealing with each of these types of statements bear more relevance for the clients with self problems who are just starting to develop more private control over "I X" statements, and less so for clients who chronically engage in destructive behaviors:

1. *Counterproductive.* Client behaviors that lead to avoidance often appear counterproductive to the therapist. For example, the second author

was supervising a case in which the client said with tears in her eyes, "I don't want to talk about my mother's death. It's just rehashing old stuff and it doesn't get me anywhere." Appropriate therapist responses would include emphasizing that she does not have to talk about it and also exploring the situation further: (a) "You look like you are about to cry, like you're really hurting inside. . . . What are you feeling? . . . Are you afraid that if you keep talking you'll start crying? . . . How did your Mom and Dad deal with you when you cried as a child?" (b) "What do you mean by 'rehashing old stuff'? . . . What's happened before when you talked about your Mom's death?" (c) "I'm feeling conflicted because I really want to respect your feelings about not talking about your Mom's death, and yet I don't want to collude in your avoiding grief feelings because I think that avoiding them is related to your avoiding close relationships in general. . . . What do you think would be more growth-enhancing for you right now—to push yourself to talk and to feel your feelings about your Mom, or to respect your feelings of not wanting to talk about her even though you know that's what I want? . . . How can we honor both your desire of not wanting to talk right now, which is important in developing your sense of self, and also your desire to make progress in therapy in general by feeling your feelings?"

2. *Self-maligning.* "I am a whore and a slut . . . I feel like the scum of the earth . . . I'm scared I'm going to become schizophrenic because my mom was." These were all statements made at different times to the second author by Ursula, a client I was seeing. My initial reaction each time was to reassure Ursula that it was not true, and each time she would get angry because she felt invalidated by me. She acknowledged that while my reassurance was important, it cut her off from describing feelings she was getting in touch with.

Gradually she trained me to combine my reassurance with allowing her the opportunity to explore her feelings: "You're definitely not a slut, but tell me all your feelings and thoughts about being a slut before I tell you why I don't think you are." "The research on schizophrenia indicates that if you haven't developed it by now, it's highly unlikely that you will. But it must be scary for you to have that fear. Tell me about it."

3. *Suicidal or homicidal.* Although suicidal and homicidal fantasies are too aversive for most therapists to listen to in any detail, it is not uncommon for clients with self problems to get in touch with these feelings because their histories are so replete with unmet needs. It is important to reinforce these expressions of feelings by helping the client

tell his or her story until the therapist thoroughly understands why it makes sense for the client to feel this way. Furthermore, it is important that the therapist forbid these harmful actions not just by mandate, but by helping the client separate feelings from actions (i.e., the connection between thinking about suicide, feeling suicidal, and engaging in suicidal behavior is that of a behavior-behavior relationship and one need not lead to the other), and by exploring in depth the consequences of suicidal or homicidal actions. If these suicidal or homicidal statements are actually mands disguised as tacts (i.e., threatening suicide because more attention is wanted from the therapist), then the client should be confronted and taught how to ask directly for what is wanted without threatening hurtful behavior.

In summary, our view of self problems focuses on early development of contingency-shaped behavior. If our notions are valid, then bringing about changes in the meaning of such core behaviors as "I love you," "I hate you," "I'm angry," and "I need attention" would seem to require a learning environment in which they can be evoked. FAP is particularly well suited for this task.

7

Functional Analytic Psychotherapy

A Bridge between Psychoanalysis and Behavior Therapy

Our radical behavioral interpretation of psychotherapy leads to the unexpected conclusion that the psychotherapeutic relationship is at the core of the therapeutic process. Unexpected, we say, because others usually cast radical behaviorism in the opposite camp, one in which the therapist avoids or discounts the value of a deep, emotional therapeutic relationship. Carl Rogers, for instance, commented, "To me [Skinner's world] would destroy the human person as I have come to know him . . . in relationship . . . in the deepest moments of psychotherapy" (1961, p. 391).

Even for those who accept that radical behaviorism can lead to an emphasis on the therapeutic relationship, they sometimes contend that functional analytic psychotherapy (FAP) adds little to what is already advocated in existing systems of therapy, and ask "so what's the big deal?" We have two reactions to this contention. First, we agree that FAP's focus on the therapeutic relationship is concordant with current trends in the field of psychotherapy. It is particularly interesting that FAP and psychoanalysis are similar in this regard because they are derived from very different philosophical and theoretical bases. Commonalities in treatment from such diverse origins are intriguing because they may indicate the universal variables that are especially important in producing therapeutic change. Second, we believe that many features of FAP are new and different. The FAP view of the therapeutic relationship and the process of change have implications for treatment that distinguish it from psychoanalysis and other therapeutic systems. In the discussion that follows, we will point out similarities and differences between FAP and psychodynamic approaches. Later, we will compare FAP with current behavior therapies and explore how it provides a unique bridge between therapy systems as divergent as psychoanalysis and behavior therapy.

FAP IN CONTRAST WITH PSYCHODYNAMIC APPROACHES

Psychoanalysis is an evolving system that comes in many forms. Its comparisons to FAP are limited to the particular ways that we characterize psychoanalysis and may not hold for other variants. The initial part of our discussion will focus on the more traditional psychodynamic views of transference and therapeutic alliance. We will then examine how a more recent form of psychoanalysis—object relations—is more compatible with FAP, yet still differs in significant ways because of its psychodynamic foundations.

Transference

To the psychoanalyst, *transference* is an important component of the client-therapist relationship. Transference is relevant to our present discussion because it refers to the client's within-session behavior. The concept, however, is "theoretically and technically burdensome and has required repeated clarification and reclarification" (Paolino, 1981, p. 91). Consequently, we will examine only a few of its central meanings, by first giving its psychoanalytic definition or description, and then by translating it into everyday language or in behavioral terms. We will then appraise how the psychoanalytic notions of transference might affect what the analyst does during the session; that is, we will look at its rule-governing features. In turn, we ask how the psychoanalyst's behavior would enable the evocation and detection of CRB1s and the reinforcement of improvements or CRB2s. Thus, even though the psychoanalyst is following the implied rules of a theory not based on behavioral concepts, we will look at the clinical implications of these rules in behavioral terms.

Freud described transference as a client's reaction to the therapist as though he or she were not him- or herself, but rather some (important) person in the client's past. He stated that this "intense emotional relationship between the [therapist] and patient," which is based on the past, arose in every analysis and that, in fact, "analysis without transference is an impossibility" (1925, p. 42).

Freud's description of transference closely resembles the behavioral concept of *stimulus generalization* (also known as *transfer*) and conveys the notion that behavior in the therapy hour is related to how a client acts in significant relationships. Furthermore, Freud considered these within-session behaviors essential for treatment and also stressed the importance of intense emotions occurring during the session. These characteristics could serve as a *rule* (see Chapter 5) which directs the analytic therapist (1) to watch for the client's emotional reactions to the therapist that also occur in other important relationships and (2) to encourage these reactions since they are essential. Positive clinical effects are likely to ensue since the behaviors called for under (1) and (2) are similar to those produced by FAP Rules 1 (Watch for CRB) and 2 (Evoke CRB).

Before looking at other meanings and the possible negative clinical effects of the concept of transference, we will discuss the behavioral concept of generalization in more detail. From a behavioral standpoint, all of our present behavior toward another person (therapist or otherwise) is based on our past learning experiences with that person and/or other people. Consequently, before there has been the opportunity to reinforce a client for a particular response, the therapist already is a stimulus which has evocative properties depending on his or her functional similarity to previous persons.

For example, after arriving late for an appointment for the first time, a client might anticipate the therapist's reactions based on previous experience with similar others. In an experiment illustrating the concept of functional similarity, Diven (1936) classically conditioned adult subjects to the stimulus word *barn* by using electric shock. When he later tested for generalization or transfer by presenting words not previously conditioned, he found that subjects showed the conditioned galvanic skin response to "cow" but not to "yarn." Transfer therefore occurred on a functional dimension (barns and cows are found on farms) and not a physical one (the phonetic similarity between "barn" and "yarn"). Thus, this particular client might anticipate the therapist's reaction to tardiness on the basis of past experiences of being late for doctors (if the functional dimension is "someone you go to for help"), or authority figures (if the functional dimension is based on "people who are in charge"), or a neglectful parent (if the functional dimension is based on "people who give insufficient time and have limited involvement"). Generalization also can be based on a combination of several functional dimensions.

From a FAP standpoint, everything a client does (says, feels, thinks, perceives, etc.) during the session are learned behaviors that occur because of (1) the functional similarity between stimuli present during the session and those present during past learning and (2) the actual experiences during therapy. This concept of within-session behaviors can account for the same phenomenon as the psychoanalytic notion of transference. Important differences between psychoanalytic and behavioral conceptions point, however, to some negative clinical implications of the concept of transference.

Defining Problematic Behavior

The concept of transference is imbued with a variety of characteristics in addition to the generalization of responses to important persons. In one of its most restrictive forms, Freud limited transference to only those within-session behaviors that are derived from certain "infantile" experiences in the Oedipal period (Langs, 1976). For example, transference narrowly referred to female clients who demanded love or friendship from their male analysts. This view of transference would result in a rule that directs the therapist to pay particular attention to within-session behavior of the Oedipal type. If a client's daily life problems just happened to be of this nature, then the therapist's sensitivity to Oedipal issues would lead to detection of CRB1 and could have positive clinical effects. Conversely, negative effects would result if the client's problems were not Oedipal, and the therapist's focus on Oedipal issues prevented him or her from noticing other kinds of CRB.

Alexander and French (1946) defined transference more broadly as "any neurotic repetition of . . . stereotyped, unsuitable, behavior based on the patient's past" which is differentiated from "normal reactions to the therapist and therapeutic situation as reality" (pp. 72-73). This rule implies that the therapist should look for behaviors that are defined as neurotic and not normal. Historically, defining abnormality has been a difficult task. In fact, interpreting the abnormality of behavior independent of its context is almost impossible. Correspondingly, the terms *neurotic, stereotyped,* and *unsuitable* all require arbitrary judgments—whether acknowledged by the therapist or not. For example, it is obvious that not all "stereotyped" behavior is transference (abnormal). The client might "stereotypically" say hello at the beginning of each session and a therapist is unlikely to judge this as transference. Similarly, the therapist must provide a context from which to judge the unsuitability of a behavior. It is possible, for instance, that a therapist could have unconscious sexist values that lead to regarding a female client's desire to pursue a career as neurotic or unsuitable.

From a FAP viewpoint, including abnormality criteria in the definition of transference creates mixed clinical effects. Such a definition could serve as a rule that leads the therapist to notice those problematic, within-session behaviors specified in the definition, and this could have positive effects if a client's daily life problems happen to be included. On the negative side, relevant behavior not included in the definition might be missed.

Even if a CRB is noticed, a more serious problem concerns such a rule's impact on the reinforcing and punishing effects of the therapist's response to the CRB. Recall that noticing a CRB helps because it is assumed that a therapist who is vigilant for and aware of the client's problematic behavior which occurs during the session, will naturally encourage and reinforce improved behavior. At times, viewing a client's response as transference would interfere with the reinforcement of improved behavior. For example, if a client historically has been compulsive in his daily life, then his repeatedly verifying appointment times could be appropriately classified as neurotic according to the definition of transference. If, however, the client historically has been remiss about keeping appointments, making schedules, and keeping track of time, then concern about appointment times would be an improvement. In this latter case, the therapist, who is guided by a fixed, noncontextual view of what is unhealthy, might offer an interpretation that inadvertently punishes the improved behavior. Because formal definitions of abnormality ignore context, the therapist views the behavior as neurotic, unsuitable, or stereotyped, and his or her natural reactions are more likely to have unintended punishing effects.

Real or Not?

For many psychoanalysts, transference involves a distortion of reality. Freud considered the client's reaction an "illusion" and thus ignored the therapist's "personality, behaviors, and role" (Langs, 1976, p. 27). A less extreme view was offered by Alexander and French (1946) who suggested that before a client reaction is classified as transference, the analyst must rule it out as a "normal reaction to the therapist and therapeutic situation as reality" (pp. 72-73). This meaning of transference could serve as a rule that directs analysts to examine their own "real" behavior and the "real" sequence of events in order to determine if the client's response is "normal" or not. In effect, this situation leads the therapist to attend to variables present in the session which affect the client's behavior. If the therapist would then share his or her observations with the client, even though this type of sharing is not usually part of psychoanalytic process, such an interaction could be beneficial because it is a description of functional relationships called for in Rule 5.

Although the real versus the transference distinction can lead therapists to examine their own contribution to the client's response, this view could have negative clinical implications because it presumes a static, single perspective (the therapist's) of reality. The "I'm right and you're wrong" outlook of reality perhaps is not problematic when a client expresses extreme accusations, such as the therapist is secretly meeting with his boss and is plotting to kill him. The "true" reality, however, is not as clear in more typical client comments such as "I don't think you care enough about me," "You are bored with me," or "Therapy costs too much money." Philosophically, there is reason to question the notion of a single, fixed truth. It is quite possible that reality can never be known (which is the radical behavioral view discussed in Chapter 1). Even if there were just one "true" reality, however, it is unreasonable to presume that the therapist will always be correct.

Clinically, we are concerned that a therapist who accepts the distorted reality aspect of transference will be less inclined to genuinely consider the possibility that a client's perception is valid when it differs from the therapist's. This, in turn, could deprive the client of an opportunity to learn how to process and resolve an interpersonal situation in which each member of the dyad has a justifiable but different view of the world. Similarly, a submissive client with an inadequate sense of self could be punished for being assertive when his or her view of reality is different from the therapist's. We have similar concerns when validation of a client's perceptions may be essential to their improvement (see Chapter 6). Such needed validation may be limited or hampered by the distorted reality notion.

We are also apprehensive that the distorted reality notion will inadvertently reinforce an authoritarian or rigid stance for therapists who are already inclined in those directions. Along these lines, psychoanalysts themselves have expressed concern that therapists might use the transference concept of "not real" to avoid real involvement with the client (Greenson, 1972). A lack of genuine involvement with the client deters the evocation of CRB and the occurrence of natural reinforcement, which is essential for therapeutic benefit in FAP.

Psychoanalysts also recognize the problems inherent in the assumption that the client's view of reality is an illusion. For example, Gill and Hoffman (1982) recently have proposed a different view of transference that is more consistent with the FAP position: "We believe that the therapist's actual behavior strongly affects the patient's actual experience, including what are usually designated as the transferential aspects of that experience. . . . We differ, therefore, from those who emphasize distortion of reality as the hallmark of the transference" (p. 139). The rule governing effects of Gill and Hoffman's view would be more likely to produce analyst behavior that resembles FAP's Rule 5.

Transference and Learned Behavior

Freud (1925) believed that transference was automatic and resulted from an inherent drive. It occurred in all cases (except if the client were psychotic) and without the therapist's "agency" (p. 42). This idea is echoed by Greenacre (1954), who conceptualized transference as a ubiquitous "primitive social instinct" (p. 672). This theory of automatic transference diverts attention from the therapist's actions that produce and maintain client reactions. In short, the roles that learning, current stimuli, and immediate reinforcement play in the therapeutic situation are abrogated. This nonlearning orientation is reflected in many psychoanalytic notions. For example, Langs (1982) described the effect of a disturbed therapist's communication as giving "patients an opportunity to place their own similar disturbances into the therapist and thereby cover their own illness with that of the therapist" (p. 136). Obviously, it is difficult to reconceptualize such notions in learning terms.

Yet, we believe that the effects of current stimuli and learning are so compelling that they must be accommodated within psychoanalysis. For instance, Waterhouse and Strupp (1984) viewed the therapist as a teacher who creates the conditions during treatment that bring about change in the client. Stone (1982) wrote that "the best 'lessons' . . . [occur] in the dyadic therapeutic relationship, i.e., on transference phenomenon. Because the latter has been witnessed by the therapist, the lesson that evolves out of its exploration will have a freshness and reality not always present in material derived from extramural life" (p. 271). The psychoanalytic position, however, does not clearly articulate what learning is, how it takes place, or its relative importance in relation to other processes. At best, it is unclear if, how, and when within-session behavior is subjected to or is the result of learning. At worst, learning is relegated to a secondary or minor role. This confusion about the role of learning produces psychoanalytic concepts that imply conflicting rules.

Consider, for example, Freud's comment that "it is impossible to destroy anyone in absentia or effigie" (1912, p. 108). Presumably, the "anyone" that Freud was referring to is the parent who was responsible for the client's dysfunctional behavior. The rest of his comment refers to the difficulty in changing this dysfunctional behavior in therapy unless the parent is once again present in the transference reaction. This notion implies the rule that it would be good for the client to react to the therapist in the same way as to a parent. To the degree that this rule encourages CRB, it has positive clinical effects. Yet, since the rule lacks any reference to learning principles, it does not give the analytic therapist much guidance on how to obtain transference reactions. The "automatic transference" assumption says the therapist need only wait for such behavior to occur.

Even worse, the absence of learning principles fosters other procedures that can interfere with the attainment of transference. An example is the principle of neutrality which asserts that "the doctor should be opaque to his patients and, like a mirror, should show them nothing but what is shown to him" (Freud, 1912, p. 118). Searles (1959) also warned against therapist emotional reactions by describing them as attempts on the therapist's part to drive a patient crazy. The implied rule is obvious—be reflective, do not react emotionally, and do not self-disclose. From a FAP viewpoint, if being opaque and nonreactive happens to make the therapist similar to a parent so that the client's problematic behavior is evoked, then it may be a good thing to do (provided the therapist is not deliberately altering his behavior so much that it brings up the dangers of arbitrary reinforcement as discussed in Chapter 1). Based on the concept of generalization, however, it is more likely that CRB involving trust, fear, love, hate, disappointment, and the like will be evoked by an involved, reactive therapist who is willing occasionally to be self-disclosing. CRB is therefore more likely to be evoked by a therapist who presents a wide range of interpersonal stimuli of the type that are likely to occur in close, meaningful relationships.

The psychoanalytic confusion regarding the role of learning can also interfere with the reinforcement process. For example, consider the principle of neutrality's effects on the reinforcing activities of the therapist. An opaque therapist's reaction would tend to be devoid of the emotion and spontaneity that often serve as reinforcers in close relationships. From a behavioral standpoint, this could be countertherapeutic because natural therapist reactions are seen as the primary change agent. According to FAP, the therapist's reactions should at times be amplified (as when the therapist has a positive reaction to the client which may be too subtle to be seen), and at other times moderated (because it can be overwhelming).

In sum, our position is that transference is operant behavior that occurs because of similarity between the present situation (which includes the therapist and the client-therapist relationship) and past ones the client has experienced. Furthermore, the therapist's reactions are contingent on client responses and will have reinforcing effects. Finally, as an operant, there is no guarantee that the problem will occur during the session. This FAP view of transference has the advantage of suggesting its causes, its relationship to the client's daily life problems, and how it is affected by the therapeutic process.

The Therapeutic Alliance

In addition to transference, *therapeutic alliance* is considered to be another important component of the client-therapist relationship. The alliance is important because it is considered to be healthy or "good," in contrast to transference which is considered neurotic or "bad." In an imprecise way, the therapeutic alliance corresponds to CRB2 and transference corresponds to CRB1. As is characteristic of all psychoanalytic concepts, there are numerous and conflicting views of therapeutic alliance. We will examine two central themes, offer a behavioral interpretation, and then look at clinical implications.

The therapeutic alliance was considered by Freud to be the primary motivating force behind treatment. It accounts for the "collaborative" aspects of the therapeutic relationship and is indistinguishable from "nonsexual, positive, transference" (Paolino, 1981, p. 100). We assume that the collaborative aspects referred to involve client behaviors, such as coming to the session even when they prefer not, talking to the therapist even when it is difficult, and following the therapist's rules even if they are considered objectionable. Furthermore, in describing these behaviors as nonsexual, they are cast as normal or healthy. In effect, an analyst following this view would have the rule-governed behavior of examining each client reaction to see if it is problematic (transference) or collaborative (alliance), and be vigilant for "good" and "bad" behavior. In turn, this would lead the analyst to react naturally to behaviors that are classified as therapeutic alliance in a positively reinforcing way, thereby strengthening them. We see this as having a positive effect because the therapist is responding, to some extent, in ways which are called for by FAP Rules 1 (Watch for CRB) and 3 (Reinforce CRB2).

Negative effects could occur, however, because of the noncontextual nature of the definition of therapeutic alliance. For example, it is conceivable that under some circumstances, a client's coming late to a session or refusing to free associate could be an improvement that needs to be reinforced. Such might be the case for an extremely passive or compulsive client, so that if the therapist interprets the noncompliant behavior as problematic because it is not therapeutic alliance, then the improvement might be punished.

The second theme characterizing therapeutic alliance revolves around a client's ability to engage in self-observation. For instance, Sterba's (1934) view of therapeutic alliance involved one of two parts of the ego. One part (defensive) is driven by instinctual and repressive forces that interfere with therapy, whereas the other part (therapeutic alliance) is realistic, seeks understanding, psychic change, and psychic growth. Similarly, Paolino (1981) described a characteristic of therapeutic alliance as "the therapist and patient agree to observe the patient's psychic functioning and behavior in an attempt to achieve a deterministic understanding of such behavior" (p. 100). These notions have as a theme the client not only acting but also standing back from and observing these actions. Furthermore, once this self-observation occurs, the client can describe what happened from a historical perspective. For example, the client might have an angry outburst at the therapist for not answering a question, but also can observe and describe the outburst as an irrational act based on how his father never answered his questions because they were considered stupid.

This second view of therapeutic alliance could function as a rule that would lead a therapist to be vigilant for, to encourage, and to naturally reinforce a client's behaviors of self-observing and describing the causes of what was self-observed. Such client behavior could have several positive clinical effects; for instance, standing back and observing oneself is part of CRB3. As described in Chapter 2, the best CRB3s involve the observation and description of one's own behavior. This same behavior enters into the formation of self-rules (Chapter 5) and the development of the self (Chapter 6). Thus, self-observation and description contribute to improvement in many aspects of one's life.

Untoward effects are possible, however, and are due to not viewing self-observing and describing as learned behaviors. For example, if they are viewed as ego functions, then the analyst's attention might be shifted to the mobilization of psychic drives involved in strengthening ego functions, rather than simply prompting and reinforcing the relevant behaviors. Second, splitting off therapeutic alliance from transference is incompatible with the notion that behavior is contextual and that alliance and transference are on the same continuum. Viewing alliance and transference as dichotomous would interfere with the natural shaping process. For example, these five behaviors are all on the same continuum: (1) "I just reacted irrationally toward you when I said I hate you," (2) "I have feelings of hating you," (3) "I hate you," (4) "Grrrr" (a sound of hating), and (5) smashing up the therapist's furniture. The first, of course, would be considered a good therapeutic alliance response. A client with a history of violent acting-out behavior, however, may have only the fifth behavior in her repertoire and may thus lack therapeutic alliance. From the FAP perspective, the occurrence of the fourth would be encouraged and reinforced as improved behavior.

Thus far we have addressed only two components of psychoanalytic theory, transference and therapeutic alliance. Other important aspects of traditional psychoanalytic theory can be summarized briefly: (1) a drive model is emphasized, where instinctual drives and libidinal impulses are our primary motivational forces; (2) the id, ego, and superego are considered to be primary structures of the human psyche; (3) the Oedipal period is emphasized; optimal psychological development is linked to occurrences that take place in the fifth or sixth year of life; (4) father occupies center stage by creating castration fear in the boy and penis envy in the girl and powerfully influences whether or not the child successfully negotiates the Oedipal period; and (5) psychopathology is related to psychosexual fixations and the inability to adequately discharge libidinal tensions (Eagle, 1984). Rather than discussing at this point how FAP is at odds with these assumptions, we will first contrast these assumptions with those of object relations theory, then compare object relations therapy with FAP. Finally, we will summarize how FAP differs from both traditional psychoanalysis and object relations theory.

Object Relations

Object relations theorists (e.g., Kernberg, 1976; Klein, 1952; Kohut, 1971; Mahler, 1952), although still considering themselves as psychoanalysts, have proposed a radical overhaul of the important aspects of traditional psychoanalytic theory that are listed above. The major differences are that in object relations theory (1) the focus is on a relational model, where human relationships are considered to be the bedrock of existence; understanding how relationships are internalized and how they become transformed into a sense of self clarifies what motivates people and how they view themselves; (2) elements of the psyche consist of relational structures (representational schema which are the internalization of relationships); (3) the pre-Oedipal period is underscored; critical events that shape people's lives are considered to take place at 5 to 6 months; (4) the interaction with mother is viewed as a template for all subsequent relationships because this initial relationship occupies so much of the early life of the child, and because it is so tied up with emotional gratification and deprivation; and (5) psychopathology centers on arrests in the development of the self and anomalies in the psychological process of splitting; since the self is interpersonally constructed, mental disturbances are tantamount to disturbances in interpersonal relationships (Cashdan, 1988).

Here is the FAP view on the five differences between traditional psychoanalysis and object relations: (1) A shift in emphasis from drives to the effects of relationships is more compatible with FAP since relationships can be translated more easily into terms of stimulus control and reinforcement. (2) Although FAP eschews explanations that focus on nonbehavioral entities, which is characteristic of all forms of psychoanalysis, the object relations view of structures as an effect of relationship experiences makes them more amenable to description in terms of external factors than does the structures of id, ego, and superego. (3) The object relations emphasis on the development of preverbal behavior could have to do with antecedents that are necessary for the development of the verbal behavior related to self (discussed in Chapter 6). A more complete behavioral analysis of self would thus incorporate these earlier experiences. There is no "critical stage" concept in FAP, however, and thus traditional and object relations views are incompatible with FAP in this respect. (4) In FAP, no particular significance is given to mothers or fathers, and caretakers are generically referred to as parents throughout the book. What is important is the nature of the specific interactions and the contingencies.

However, some features of the object relations position make it more compatible to FAP. First, the notions of gratification and deprivation are closer to the behavioral concepts of reinforcement and deprivation and are thus more easily translated into environmental events. Second, gratification and deprivation are more abstract notions of motivation than castration and penis envy and thus are more similar to reinforcement (a very abstract conception of motivation). Finally, although we disagree with the conclusion that the mother is always most important, the argument that the child is shaped by the one who delivers the most contingencies is consistent with the FAP position. (5) The object relations concept of splitting (viewing the self or someone else as all good at one time and as all bad at another) is presented as a process and lends itself more easily to interpretation involving behavioral processes (such as seeing under discriminative control and remembering) than such concepts as psychosexual fixations and the discharge of libidinal tensions. The isomorphism between mental states and interpersonal states similarly draws attention to the external variables that constitute an interpersonal relationship.

In view of the greater compatibility of object relations concepts with FAP, it would be anticipated that clinical process might also be more compatible. As expected, the description by Cashdan (1988) of object relations therapy bears a striking resemblance to FAP:

> Of the various relationships that make up the patient's life, prime considera-
> tion would be given to the relationship with the therapist. Not only does it
> occur in the phenomenological here-and-now, but it also contains many of
> the critical elements operative in the patient's relationships with others. The
> therapist-client relationship consequently would be viewed as an *in vivo* ex-
> pression of what is pathological in the patient's life. If this were the case, it
> would be reasonable to conclude that the therapist-patient relationship con-
> tains the greatest potential for change. Rather than being viewed as a means
> of producing insight, self-awareness, or other changes "in the patient," the
> therapist-patient relationship *itself* would become the focus of change. (p. 28)

Striking similarities notwithstanding, Cashdan's object relations therapy reveals some marked divergences from FAP. For example, his focus is on the patient's psychological mechanism of *projective identification*, a pattern of interpersonal behavior in which the patient manipulates others to behave or respond in a circumscribed fashion. Projective identifications distort and undermine the patient's current relationships and represent "maladaptive efforts to redress the goodness-badness balance of the inner world" (p. 56), which comes from unsatisfactory object relations that are largely historical in nature. Thus, the individual "unconsciously projects a part of the self into another human being as a means of converting an inner struggle over badness and unacceptability into an external one" (p. 57). According to Cashdan, major projective identifications include dependency (induces caretaking in others), power (induces feelings of weakness and incompetency in others), sexuality (induces sexual arousal), and ingratiation (self-sacrifice, which induces others to be grateful).

Needless to say, this profusion of mental entities is not consistent with a FAP approach. Looking at the projective identification of dependency, we would view it in these ways: (1) Nothing is projected into someone else; the client is acting dependent because he or she was reinforced for it in the past, and was probably punished as a child for exhibiting more independent behaviors. (2) No conversion of an inner struggle into an outer one takes place; the inner struggle is a side effect of both dependent and independent responses having been punished at different times. (3) Being this dependent has lost much of its past adaptive value; dependence now constitutes an avoidance behavior that prevents the client from contacting more positive contingencies associated with building in new behaviors (e.g., being assertive, taking control, having the ability to give and take).

More importantly, in terms of clinical implications, we view the designation of specific behaviors (i.e., dependence, power, sexual, ingratiation) as projective identifications to be problematic. There is an *a priori* judgment that if a therapist responds to the client's behavior with feelings of caretaking, incompetence, sexual arousal or gratefulness, it is a reflection of the client's pathology and is therefore undesirable. As we have repeatedly stated, behaviors cannot be judged as problematic without considering the larger context; that is, although these client behaviors might be problematic (CRB1s), it is also possible that they are improvements (CRB2s) when considering the client's current repertoire. For instance, if a female client generally avoided relationships because she was afraid of being too dependent, then an emergence of dependence behavior would actually be a CRB2 and should be reinforced in the earlier stages of the therapy. Or, if dependence had been agreed upon as a CRB1, then improvements need to be shaped and reinforced rather than punished. An improvement might be the client's calling the therapist only once or twice a week as opposed to four or five times a week, or shortening her lengthy phone conversations to less than 10 minutes. The object relations view of the behavior as pathological might lead to the punishment of dependency behaviors, which are an improvement over previous ones.

In sum, although some features of object relations are more compatible with the radical behavioral view than is traditional psychoanalysis, both object relations and the traditional psychoanalytic view share fundamental assumptions that are at odds with FAP. These are (1) mentalistic structures cause behavior (both adaptive and maladaptive), (2) our basic personalities are formed through important interactions with either the father or mother during specific critical developmental periods, and (3) specific behaviors of the client (e.g., splitting, projective identifications) are given *a priori* status as pathological. In contrast, FAP (1) focuses on environmental events as the ultimate causes of behavior, (2) holds that important events shape our behavior throughout our lifetimes, and (3) emphasizes the contextual meaning of behavior—that the same behavior may be pathological or adaptive depending on the context in which it occurs.

FAP IN CONTRAST WITH CURRENT BEHAVIOR THERAPIES

FAP differs from other behavior therapies primarily in the core significance given to certain aspects of the therapeutic relationship. Specifically, FAP stresses that the therapeutic relationship is an environment that can evoke and immediately consequate clinically relevant behavior. Rarely has this aspect of the relationship been mentioned by behavior therapists. Some notable exceptions include Goldfried and Davison (1976), who pointed out that within-session behavior could, at times, be useful in the process of behavior therapy. Also, Goldfried (1982) pointed to the client-therapist relationship as central to the understanding of resistance during behavior therapy. The therapeutic opportunity of client problems occurring within the session was also recognized by Goldfried, who saw resistance as "a mixed blessing in that [it] interfere[s] with the course of therapy but at the same time provide[s] the therapist with a firsthand sample of the client's problem" (p. 105). Even though these authors acknowledged the occurrence of client problems during the session and their potential role in treatment, they also saw them as playing a relatively minor role in the methods of behavior therapy. Further, their views seem to have had little impact in the field. Instead, when behavior therapists talk about the therapeutic relationship and recognize its importance, they typically refer to such factors as "nonspecific effects," "the using of a 'good relationship' as the basis for obtaining cooperation during treatment" or "using the therapist's social reinforcement value to motivate or maintain changes in daily life." As important as such variables are, they do not direct attention, as does FAP, to the clinically relevant behaviors occurring during the session.

This difference in focus is clear in Sweet's (1984) review of therapeutic relationship issues attended to by behavior therapists that include such factors as impact of the relationship, therapist time, and social reinforcement. None of the reviewed studies mentioned the importance of the client's presenting problem behaviors that occur during the session. Sometimes, these behaviors were ignored even though they attracted the attention of the therapist as in this case example given by Sweet. He described how a client was frightened of making progress in treatment which was manifested, in part, by her negative reactions to the therapist's praise (social reinforcement was the therapeutic procedure being employed). The therapist used flooding to "overcome this impasse." In citing this case as an example of overcoming a technical difficulty, "fear of success," in doing the therapy, Sweet overlooked the potential importance of the "fear of success" in the therapeutic relationship as an occurrence of a problem that had significant impact in other areas of this client's life. Furthermore, no consideration was given to the potential benefits that the "overcoming of a technical difficulty" may have had for the client in her daily life.

FAP is similar to social skills training because it emphasizes deficits in interpersonal repertoires as the cause of the client's problems and views treatment as a means of remediating the deficits. The techniques differ markedly, however, in how the skill deficits are detected and in the remediation process itself. In FAP, the therapist is directed to observe, during the session, actual occurrences of presenting symptoms and the variables controlling them. Targeting the type and amount of behavioral improvement is based on the particular client's existing repertoire. Such target behaviors might be subtle and difficult to recognize without this direct observation. For example, this situation was true with Agnes (the client discussed earlier), whose improvement consisted of giving reasons for quitting therapy before actually doing it. In FAP, perhaps most importantly, an improvement is a behavioral change that occurs under the stimulus conditions which bring about the symptoms. In fact, the functional equivalence between the therapeutic situation and the natural environment is a precondition for FAP. If the therapeutic situation does not evoke the symptoms, FAP cannot be done. Thus, in the FAP system, symptoms and improvements are functionally defined.

In contrast, social skills training rarely involves the direct observation of the symptoms or the conditions that bring them about. Furthermore, the skills are acquired under conditions that are obviously different from the conditions that bring about the symptoms. Behavior acquired via coaching, modeling, role-playing, and behavioral rehearsal during the session is functionally different from the behavior that is supposed to occur in daily life even though they might look the same. Ignoring the functional aspects of the behavior is like ignoring the difference between rote learning the sounds that comprise a sentence in French and learning the same sounds with an understanding of their meaning. The sentences may sound exactly the same to a listener but they are functionally very different. An allusion to this problem can be found in a review of the literature on social skills training generalization by Scott, Himadi, and Keane (1983). They concluded that the lack of demonstrable generalization is responsible for social skill training's limited acceptability as a viable treatment. From a FAP viewpoint, the lack of functional similarity between training and natural environments that typifies social skills training provides no guarantee that trained behavior will transfer and that explanations are needed to account for those instances in which it does.

Differences notwithstanding, it should be emphasized that FAP complements and overlaps with other behavior therapies. Since behavior therapy has demonstrated its effectiveness, it still is the treatment of choice for initial intervention in most situations. In contrast, the empirical data to support the efficacy of FAP have not yet been gathered. For this reason alone, it makes sense to try behavior therapy as the first intervention and then to complement it with FAP as the occasion or need arises.

FAP was developed in the context of ongoing behavior therapy. At first, it was used when behavior therapy appeared to be ineffective. Now, we use FAP in conjunction with behavior therapy from the very beginning, and at times, it becomes the primary mode of treatment. FAP is easily integrated with behavior therapy because many of the methods of behavior therapy are evocative of CRB. For example, specific homework instructions are often assigned during behavior therapy. For clients whose problems involve excessive compliance, rebelliousness, or guilt or anxiety for not meeting expectations, these assignments naturally provide an opportunity for FAP.

FAP: A UNIQUE NICHE BETWEEN PSYCHOANALYSIS AND BEHAVIOR THERAPY

The methods of FAP overlap those of behavioral and of psychoanalytic therapies. To illustrate this position, let us consider the case of Melissa, aged 29, who came into therapy with the second author for recurring depression and distress about her "poor self-worth." Her everyday functioning was not going well, and she felt like she was "drowning." Feeling no enthusiasm for life, she admitted seriously contemplating suicide. She struggled with questions of, "Am I worthwhile? Can I forgive myself? Am I really worthy of being loved?" We noted that she had never been in an intimate relationship. Behavioral treatments have traditionally avoided these difficult-to-specify problems and have left them to psychodynamically oriented therapists. Yet, we have argued that these types of client problems do lend themselves to a behavioral analysis.

Many of the repertoires to be shaped were those needed for intimate relating. Furthermore, many of Melissa's CRB1s were evoked only by long-term relationships. Thus, the treatment, too, was long-term—I saw Melissa over a 5-year period. The length of her treatment resembled the length of psychoanalytic treatments, yet the rationale is behavioral.

In our opinion, the outcome was excellent. At the end of 5 years, Melissa was in a committed relationship and wrote the following description of therapy: "What [the therapist] helped me to do was give myself time to heal from all the pain. She listened to me, she comforted me, she loved me, unconditionally. And as a result of giving myself that time and letting this person love me, I have a life of abundant love and hope, beyond anything I ever dreamed of before." We are in favor of the rigorous evaluations characteristic of behavioral treatments and offer the above outcome evaluation as an interim method. Like psychoanalysis, however, FAP is a complex and longer term treatment that does not easily lend itself to traditional outcome evaluation.

My stance in the therapy with Melissa was to be a "real" person with whom Melissa could engage and struggle. That is, I did not hide my emotions, my opinions, my values behind a "blank screen." Because of this, I evoked the problems that she had in forming and maintaining a close relationship. However, I also provided in therapy the opportunity for new behavior to emerge and to be reinforced. The following are a few of the specific interactions reflecting the process that resulted in Melissa's improvement:

Excerpt 1

C: I'm always nervous around you. I'm telling you about my life, my feelings, I feel naked. When I don't tell, I feel safe. When I do, I can't predict me or you. I'm worried about what you'll think. (This is a significant CRB2 since Melissa rarely reported her feelings. Client reports of this nature are encouraged by FAP and psychoanalysis.)

T: I feel closer to you when you let me know who you are. (I am amplifying a private response which is a potential natural reinforcer. While this is generally viewed as countertherapeutic by psychoanalysts and not usually done by behavior therapists, it is advisable to do according to the FAP rules.)

C: I haven't ever felt my feelings so close to the surface before, felt them so acutely. (Rule 4 suggests observation of the effects of reinforcement. This response appears to reflect an immediate result of the reinforcing effects of the therapist's response.)

Excerpt 2

T: What will it be like not seeing me for 4 weeks? (A focus on the effects of the therapist's going on vacation is standard fare in FAP and in psychoanalysis. Although not usually attended to by behavior therapists, FAP offers a behavioral rationale for doing so in some cases.)

C: Hard, cause I feel attached to you. This is the one place where I can say, do, cry, as I please. An upside to not seeing you for a month is that it's a chance for me to practice being more intimate with people I care about. (This is a CRB2, an important response for both FAP and psychoanalysis.)

T: I'm going to miss you, too. (This is good to do in FAP but generally is a no-no in psychoanalysis.)

Excerpt 3

C: I have shut myself off from almost everyone and it's intentional. I'm going down and I don't want to pull them down with me. I don't want to be a burden.

T: Do you feel that way about me? (Behavior therapists might have challenged her irrational idea of being a burden and would not have asked about her feelings about me. Psychoanalysts would probably have done what I did. FAP would, at times, call for either.)

Excerpt 4

T: You've really opened up to me, to yourself, and to others. You've gotten yourself out of suicidal periods, you're learning more about what gets you in and out of these moods, taking more risks, learning more about what you want, what you're feeling and how to talk about these feelings. You're clearer about your sexuality. . . . (This is an interpretation which has features of interest to both psychoanalysts and behavior therapists. The comparison between her within-session behavior and the behavior occurring in daily life is characteristic of psychoanalysis. The emphasis on the functional relationship between her behavior and mood in daily life is more characteristic of behavior therapy. FAP interpretations contain elements of both.)

T: What are you feeling right now?

C: Nothing. [with *a sneering look on her face*]

T: It feels like a slap in the face, you know. (This comment is a within-session contingency which blocked her avoidance. Psychoanalysts would have noted her behavior but probably not have blocked the avoidance with a personal statement.)

C: Why?

T: I've been telling you what I think, you must have some reactions to it, but you say "nothing" with a sneer on your face and I don't know what's going on. (While I am attending to her within-session behavior as suggested by psychoanalysis, the interpretation is based on behavioral principles.)

C: I'll be back in a few minutes. . . . (She leaves and returns.) I just shut down, got really scared. The biggest thing this year is how I've let you into my life. I've never felt so supported in such a deep and consistent level by anyone before. It's scary to tell you. (Note that this is a CRB2.)

T: It makes me feel closer to you when you tell me things that are scary. (Again, this is an amplification of a personal response which serves as a natural reinforcer.)

Other types of interventions I made included directly helping Melissa in her employment-seeking activities by critiquing her resume, reviewing her job applications, role-playing interviews, and teaching her relaxation skills to help with interview anxiety. All of these activities are standard fare for behavior therapists but are avoided by psychoanalysts. FAP provides a rationale for how and when the behavior therapy approach is appropriate as well as for when psychoanalytic passivity would be more effective.

In sum, we hope that FAP can address the shortcomings and yet include the best aspects of both psychoanalysis and behavior therapies. The benefits and drawbacks of integration of behavioral and psychoanalytic approaches have been discussed by Messer (1983, 1986). For some, the drawbacks are the compromises called for by integrating behavior therapy's emphasis on scientific precision, parsimony, and melioration with the psychoanalytic emphasis on open-ended exploration and the understanding of cognitions, behavior, and affect. With further development, FAP appears to offer a means for integration that could minimize these compromises.

8

Reflections on Ethical, Supervisory, Research, and Cultural Issues

In this final chapter, we will discuss some of the ethical issues involved in the conduct of functional analytic psychotherapy (FAP). We will then describe how the principles of FAP can be applied to the supervisory process. Then, we turn our attention to the important question of "Where are the data" and our somewhat unconventional ideas of how to go about collecting these data. Finally, for something really different, we will discuss such topics as fast food, spirituality, and how the principles underlying FAP can be broadened to address the problems facing our culture in general.

ETHICAL ISSUES

Codes such as the *Ethical Principles of Psychologists* (APA, 1981) and books like *Ethics in Psychology* (Keith-Spiegel & Koocher, 1985) offer professional standards intended to guide clinicians in ethical conduct. To augment these guidelines (rules), we have selected a number of issues for further discussion.

Before proceeding, however, we have a few words about the behavioral perspective on ethics, based, in part, on Zuriff (1987) and Skinner (1974). A given event can serve as a reinforcer for (1) the client's behavior, (2) the therapist's behavior, (3) the well-being of the members of the professional group, (4) the well-being of members of the larger society, and

(5) the survival of the culture. Ethical problems occur when long-term reinforcers are positive for one or more of these five groups, but not for all.
Later, in a section on cultural problems, we will touch on the issue of
individual reinforcement conflicting with the survival of culture. Although
not discussed here, some of the APA ethical guidelines and Keith-Spiegel
and Koocher address conflicting contingencies for the individual therapist
and the professional group. In fact, Keith-Spiegel and Koocher's definition
of ethics, a set of guidelines for conduct essential in "maintaining the in-
tegrity and cohesiveness of a profession" (1985, p. xiii), emphasizes the
importance of reinforcers for the professional group in general. We believe,
however, that therapist and client contingencies which conflict are the most
important source of ethical problems. Accordingly, we have focused on
these issues in this section and in our discussions of arbitrary reinforcement
in Chapter 1 and Rule 3 in Chapter 3.

Since clients often come to us in pain and in need of comfort and
guidance, they are particularly susceptible to the influence of the therapist. Psychotherapists are in a position to help effect great change at
such vulnerable times in clients' lives, but conversely, the potential for
great harm also exists. The issues we raise are relevant to therapists of
any theoretical orientation, but some are particularly relevant to FAP
because of the potency of its procedures. We will discuss some precautions to help minimize the possibility that FAP will be misused to abuse
or exploit clients.

Proceed Cautiously

The controlling variables that occur during the therapy session can
be very potent. FAP procedures tend to evoke intense emotional reactions and reinforcing effects that are associated with intimate relationships. Because of this, FAP can be very beneficial to the client by affecting
large repertoires. For example, during FAP, a client could learn for the
first time to trust another human being. These same within-session controlling variables, however, can be extremely aversive and produce
harmful effects for the client, such as intense negative affect and associated avoidance and escape repertoires. Thus, a client might quit therapy
and become a hermit because the "letting down of one's guard" that
happens when a person trusts can evoke avoidance, escape, and accompanying pain.

Since it is common for CRB1 to be aversively controlled behavior,
it is often necessary to have some aversiveness present in order to (1)
evoke the CRB that is required for FAP and (2) block the ensuing avoidance. Although too little aversiveness hampers progress because the cli-

ent's avoidance is successfully reinforced in the session, too much aversiveness can overwhelm and immobilize. Clients whose behavior is frequently disrupted by reactions to aversive stimuli should be exposed to FAP procedures with caution. For example, consider a client who was extremely sensitive to criticism. In one instance, he was emotionally devastated and missed several days of work because a co-worker criticized him for a minor error. FAP would, at first, be used sparingly with this client since a focus on within-session behavior might lead to a hint of criticism, which, in turn, could be overwhelming for him if it occurred in the here and now. Generally, it is a good idea to start treatment with a focus on problems that occur outside the session using procedures from other therapy systems before doing anything about CRB; that is, before focusing on the therapist-client relationship. This procedure will help to develop the task orientation of treatment and give both client and therapist a chance to establish a general method of working together without complications from disruptive emotional reactions. Proceeding cautiously also means that identifying a within-session behavior as CRB is a hypothesis to be explored, and the actual clinical relevance needs to be demonstrated, not assumed.

Avoid Sexual Exploitation

Because focusing on behavior that occurs during the session intensifies the feelings between client and therapist, sexual attraction between the two individuals may result. Even though discussion of such feelings can provide opportunities for therapeutic progress, acting on them is countertherapeutic and unethical. A similar issue is involved when a client has sexual problems. A naive or self-serving therapist may argue that according to the tenets of FAP, the best intervention would be to become sexual with the client since the clinically relevant behaviors would only come up in a sexual relationship. Rather, in such a situation, sex therapy with the client and a significant other would be the best intervention. Because sex between client and therapist seems to be arbitrarily reinforced by the therapist, the client sooner or later feels exploited and betrayed. This is confirmed by the increasing number of malpractice suits brought by clients against therapists who have had sex with them.

Guard against the Continuation of a Nonbeneficial Treatment

The basic FAP notion that CRB occurs within the therapeutic relationship may result in the continuation of a nonbeneficial treatment. For example, a client whose problems center on not being able to terminate destructive relationships may also show similar behavior during a non-helpful therapy. Therefore, a client may stay in therapy when it would be better if treatment were terminated, or if the client were referred to another therapist. Furthermore, the role of the therapist as expert/authority figure decreases the likelihood that the client will take the initiative to terminate, particularly when he or she has been cautioned against leaving treatment prematurely.

Be Aware of Prejudicial and Oppressive Values

Because of its radical behavioral foundations, FAP does not have any sexist, racist, or otherwise discriminatory assumptions; specifically, there are no models of what a healthy person should be like or what kinds of goal behaviors should be in his or her repertoire. What is favored are positively reinforced repertoires and an eschewing of aversive controls. There is, therefore, no theoretical basis for deciding what specific behaviors should be in the repertoires of a person based on race, gender, sexual orientation, age, physical disabilities, or membership in any other group. The theory is neutral with respect to these issues.

The therapist, however, as a member of the culture that supports subtle, and sometimes not so subtle, forms of prejudice and discrimination could have values consistent with the culture. Values refer to a person's reinforcers; this means that a sexist or racist therapist would continue to reinforce those client behaviors that have been shaped by a racist or sexist culture. We believe the most deleterious effect of oppression is that access to reinforcers is limited. For example, a woman who has learned always to acquiesce because of sexist training will not have access to reinforcers that require assertiveness. Similarly, a male who was punished for showing feelings and who thus avoids evocative situations, will not have access to reinforcers available in an intimate relationship that requires the expressing of feelings. Needless to say, access to reinforcement is limited when educational, employment, and relationship opportunities are denied on the basis of race, gender, or other minority group membership. Consequently, a therapist who reinforces on the basis of sexism or racism would be interfering with repertoires that could increase long-term positive reinforcement and thereby compromise the goals of FAP. This problem is compounded by the fact that the bias may be subtle and not self-observable by the therapist. As a precaution against such bias, it is helpful to have sessions regularly videotaped and observed by individuals who are sensitive to such issues.

Avoid Emotional Tyranny

Emotional tyranny is a term used by Jeffrey Masson (1988) to describe abuses of power by psychotherapists to the detriment of their clients. According to Masson, abuse is built into the very fabric of psychotherapy because of the power imbalance between client and therapist. The therapist's power extends to the structure of the therapy session, how long it lasts, how often it occurs, what is and is not permissible behavior within the session, and how much it costs. Masson also doubted the value of a therapeutic relationship based on the therapist's warmth, attention, and concern, because these qualities can only be ascribed to someone a person knows in an equal relationship. Psychotherapy, Masson concluded (p. 251), is "a profession that depends for its existence on other people's misery," and is by its very nature, flawed and corrupt.

The mental, emotional, physical, and sexual abuses committed within the profession, which were documented by Masson, are frightening and sobering, and his allegations of the flawed and corrupt nature of psychotherapy require rigorous self-scrutiny on the part of clinicians. We will examine some of the major arguments of his critique, describe a FAP view of emotional tyranny, and suggest ways to limit the abuse of power by our profession.

First, the practical matter as to whether or not the abuses are offset, on balance, by the good effects of psychotherapy is a social value question. The answer to this question will be based largely on empirical findings regarding the number and the severity of bad effects compared to the number and the quality of good effects. As an aside, it appears that Masson's bias seriously compromises his evaluation of the empirical question. For example, he used individual patient reports as evidence for abuses while, at the same time, viewed individual client reports that support the value of therapy ("I would be dead without her help" [p. 241]) as a myth.

Second, Masson implied that a "real" relationship can occur only when it is equal. This requirement for reality seems overly restrictive. In the real world, real relationships are equal in some respects and unequal in others. From a FAP standpoint, the realness of the relationship is functionally defined. If it evokes such genuine feelings as anger, love or terror, then something "real" has occurred. Equality along some dimension is not a necessary condition for something real to occur.

Third, in terms of the power imbalance, our view is that such imbalances cannot be said to be therapeutically good, bad, or neutral without knowing the context. Whether a power imbalance is therapeutic or not depends on the nature of the client's problem and the contingent responses of the therapist. If the client's problem is evoked by a power difference, then the power difference that occurs in therapy could be a necessary (but not sufficient) condition for successful treatment. Consider, for example, a client who has been unable to assert himself and has been taken advantage of by people who have power over him (like bosses, police, the IRS, editors, and teachers). Since he has been unable to learn new ways of relating to authorities in the natural environment, therapy can provide an ideal learning opportunity for this client because the power difference is similar to the natural environment. In the treatment environment, the client's assertiveness and independence could be strengthened if the therapist were reinforced by such improvements. If, however, the therapist fails to do this and, instead, reinforces the powerlessness of the client, then abuse has taken place.

From a FAP standpoint, the major way that abuse can occur with therapy is when a therapist's actions are controlled by reinforcers other than the client's progress. For example, in private practice, the therapist's fees are contingent on keeping the client in therapy which, in turn, might be countertherapeutic. More problematic than money, however, are other conceivable therapist reinforcers, such as the client's subservience, admiration, civility, flirtatiousness, masculinity, femininity, and the like. Just because these reinforcers could be responsible for the therapist's behavior does not mean that they are. Nevertheless, the problem is difficult to solve.

In light of the potential for abuse, outside monitoring of the therapy process by peers and supervisors using audiotapes and videotapes seems important in preventing this type of abuse. Such monitoring, of course, is subject to the consent of the client involved. Furthermore, ways should be found to ensure that practicing therapists (1) are well-trained, clinically aware, and sensitive; (2) have the client's requisite behaviors in their own repertoires; and (3) be the kind of people who are likely to be reinforced by client improvements and not by other reinforcers that are countertherapeutic. FAP supervision (discussed next) applies the principles of FAP to the supervisory relationship, and can aid in ensuring the suitability of therapists for FAP.

FAP SUPERVISION

The FAP supervisor first explains the rules of FAP didactically in much the same way that they were presented in this book. Then, the supervisor helps to put the rules into practice by viewing the therapy sessions and offering FAP interpretations of the client-therapist interaction. Direct observation behind a one-way mirror is the most preferred mode of accessing the supervisee's work; videotapes and audiotapes of the sessions are also used. The effectiveness of FAP supervision is greatly enhanced, however, if the CRB relevant to the client-therapist interaction can be brought into the supervisor-supervisee relationship.

For example, the second author was supervising a graduate student whose client had difficulties in self-concept and in expressing her feelings when these supervisory interactions took place:

Supervisor: I'm excited about working with you. I think you're really special, and I feel a sense of familiarity and comfort with you that's rare with someone I don't know very well.

Supervisee: I'm really excited too. I left our last meeting feeling this warm glow inside, and decided to just let myself feel it for as long as I could. I was telling my friends that this is the way graduate school should be.
(Several months later.)

Supervisor: What are the parallels and differences between our process and you and your client's?

Supervisee: She and I are both reserved, and working on being present. The differences are that my relationship with her feels more constrained, I'm sure by me, but I feel like it's constrained by her. I get pulled into people's ways of being pretty easily. I want to remain myself, more constant. With you, I have feelings of closeness and I don't know what to do about it.

Supervisor: I feel the same way. I don't know that we have to do anything about our feelings of closeness. I have a tendency to get intensely involved in relationships too quickly, so I'd like to just sit back and feel the closeness between us, enjoy it, talk about it, and see what happens over time.

These interactions show how the supervisory relationship can be a model for the therapist-client relationship; that is, not only is the supervisee-client relationship a focus, but priority is also placed on the relationship between the supervisee and the supervisor. The collegial nature of the affiliation brings an added dimension to the relationship, and a mutual sharing can take place between supervisor and supervisee that usually would not be possible, nor called for, with a client.

Since the therapy session for this student therapist's client usually began with the client's reporting how she felt and what had happened during the week, we often would start the supervisory session by talking about what we were feeling at the moment and issues we were thinking about and struggling with. Then, needless to say, the client's clinically relevant behaviors and the principles of FAP became the focal points of discussion. Some typical questions asked of the supervisee include:

1. How are you feeling about this supervision session? How do you feel about the feedback I've given you? What do you want more of from me? Less of? (These questions are parallel to those asked of the client by the therapist.)
2. When your client talks about things that you think are irrelevant, what kinds of multiple causation could be operating which convey subtle concerns of the client? How can you use your feelings of anger and boredom as discriminative stimuli to help you be a better therapist with her?
3. What are you feeling toward me? What are your fears and expectations about our relationship? (These are parallel to the questions asked of the client by the therapist.)
4. Are there any similarities between your client's issues and your own?
5. I noticed that you do not appear different when your client cries. What do you feel when she's crying? What are your own feelings about crying?
6. I'd like you to make a list of what you feel is okay to want from me in this relationship, and what you feel isn't okay to want. (This request paralleled an assignment the supervisee was to give her client.)

Thus, in supervision, not only is FAP taught didactically, but, more importantly, it is taught experientially. The supervisory relationship is difficult and challenging, and yet rewarding, for the student therapist who is required to develop intimacy skills, to be open, vulnerable, honest, aware, and present. Even though topics may sometimes overlap what is covered in personal therapy, supervision is distinct from therapy because the focus is on the development of the supervisee's clinical skills, and there is not a sustained focus on the supervisee's personal issues, but rather an exploration of how these personal issues impact his or her work.

RESEARCH AND EVALUATION

The behaviorist's commitment to the collection of data is well known. So the question can be asked, "Are there any systematic outcome or process data to support FAP?" Regrettably, at this time, there are no data of this type. FAP is informed, however, by an abundance of data from laboratory studies on such basic concepts as reinforcement, avoidance, stimulus control, and rules. But since we have extended these concepts into areas that far exceed the laboratory conditions, FAP has the status of a hypothesis.

Many specific subhypotheses implicit in FAP can be tested empirically. For example, it is hypothesized that outcome is enhanced if (1) the therapy is structured to evoke occurrences during the session of the client's clinically relevant behavior; (2) the therapist notices client's problem-relevant and goal-related behaviors as they occur during the session; (3) the therapist has the goal-related repertoires in her or his repertoire; (4) the therapist's reactions shape and naturally reinforce client improvements; and (5) the therapist offers interpretations about the client's behavior that include discriminative stimuli, the behavior being interpreted, and reinforcement. These subhypotheses could be evaluated by using a traditional research strategy involving at least two groups of randomly assigned subjects, one of which would receive FAP while the other would not. Variations of this traditional research strategy might involve additional control groups and the assessment of within-group comparisons, subject factors, therapist factors, and type of problem being treated.

A number of practical considerations, however, make it nearly impossible to use the traditional research approach. For example, FAP is a lengthy treatment that requires intensive training for therapists. Thus, the time and resources needed to complete such a study would be formidable. Since FAP is still in its early developmental stages, the commitment of extensive resources to such a study would be unjustified and premature. Even if these obstacles could be overcome, there is reason to question the usefulness of this type of research strategy for our present purposes. In the sections that follow, we will survey the pitfalls of traditional research paradigms and suggest alternative methods for collecting data to influence clinical practice.

Pitfalls of Traditional Research Paradigms

In examining the problems associated with traditional research design, we first ask the question, "What is the purpose of clinical research?" From a functional perspective, we are asking, "What are the contingencies that maintain a researcher's use of particular research methods?" Although social contingencies include requirements for publication, advancement to tenure, and acceptance by other researchers and granting agencies, the main reason clinical researchers do what they do is to discover improved methods of treatment that are integrated into clinical practice. Thus, the practicing clinician is the consumer of clinical research. Whether or not the researcher's products are used by the practitioner is the ultimate reinforcer that supposedly maintains the researcher's activities.

What is supposed to be and what actually happens, however, are not the same thing. According to Barlow, a distinguished clinical researcher, "clinical research has little or no influence on clinical practice" (1981, p. 147). This is true even for practicing behavioral clinicians. How can this be? Our discipline has had the goal of integrating science and practice for the last 30 years, and untold millions of dollars have been spent doing the research. The root of the problem, according to Barlow, lies in the limitations of traditional research strategies involving group comparison research.

The requirements of doing this type of research often preclude the possibility that practicing clinicians can use the obtained results. For example, inferential statistics, a hallmark of traditional research, has been quite problematic. In order to obtain statistically significant results, researchers must keep between-subject variability to a minimum by selecting a group of subjects who are as similar as possible. This means that certain categories of subjects are excluded, such as those who (1) are too young, (2) are too old, (3) are male (or female), (4) are on medication, (5) have difficulty speaking English, (6) have emotional problems in addition to the one being studied, or (7) have serious chronic health problems.

Furthermore, inferential statistical analyses require large numbers of subjects. Thus, the only clinical problems that are studied are those which are accessible in large numbers. Traditional research is facilitated if a specific, objective problem, such as agoraphobia or sexual dysfunction, is studied since reliable outcome measures are available. Often, research subjects must be willing to wait for treatment, to collect data, to understand and sign a complex consent form, to be seen by student therapists, to commit to completing a course of treatment, to read English, to not be suicidal, and so forth. Since the clients seen in clinical practice are unselected, rarely are they the same as those used in traditional research.

Correspondingly, the results obtained may not apply to clients seen in practice. In clinical practice, clients often present vague, subjective, multiple complaints. Since research subjects tend to have specific, objective problems and information on individual subjects is not available, the clinician cannot find studies on the problems seen in practice. In a word, traditional research strategies produce information that is not relevant to clinical practice.

Another criticism of traditional research strategies is that they do not lead to innovation in theory or treatment (Mahrer, 1988). Thus, another reason clinicians do not use research findings in practice is that they contribute little that is new. It is to the credit of traditional research methodologists that they are engaging in self-examination which calls their methods into question (Barlow, 1981; Greenberg & Pinsof, 1986; Rice & Greenberg, 1984). The alternatives, however, are less clear. In the next section, we will deal with this problem functionally by looking at what does influence practice, and then making generalizations about the data involved.

Alternative Methods of Data Collection That Influence Clinical Practice

Personal clinical experience is probably near the top of every therapist's list in terms of what influences his or her clinical behavior. Joseph Matarazzo, a prominent clinical researcher, stated that "even after 15 years, few of my research findings affect my practice. Psychological science per se doesn't guide me one bit. I still read avidly, but this is of little direct practical help. *My clinical experience is the only thing that has helped me in my practice to date*" (italics added) (cited in Bergin & Strupp, 1972, p. 340).

Several factors give personal experience its strong influence. Most importantly, the clinician is exposed to a mass of raw data: all that has been said, the client's tone of voice, his or her facial expressions, posture, grimaces, and motor activity as well as such external conditions as weather, international crises, flu epidemics, and so forth. To be sure, the raw data are subject to the biases (seeing and remembering behavior) of the clinician, but our impression is that clinicians remember a surprisingly large amount of detailed information over the time span of a client's therapy. Perhaps such a large amount of information is retained because of the clinician's involvement in the process, which is comparable to the remembering that each of us has for details and major events throughout the course of our lives.

Whatever amount is personally seen and remembered by a clinician about an individual's therapy vastly exceeds the amount of data that are contained in the ratings, scales, test results, and descriptions given in even the most detailed and comprehensive traditional research reports. This extremely large number of observations has some important advantages.

First, it sensitizes the therapist to trends and base rates for a large number of variables, which, in turn, facilitate assessments of change. For example, genuine laughing by a client during a therapy session may be a marked and significant change noticed by the therapist even though the absence of laughing was not previously a focus of attention. In effect, as therapy progresses, the therapist is collecting baseline data on a large number of variables so that the detection of significant changes is made possible. Such changes would be missed in the traditional research study because data are collected on only a limited number of preselected variables.

Second, there is a cornucopia of information about the client's history, daily life interactions, and other characteristics that are based on initial interviews and an ongoing therapeutic relationship. As the therapist gains experience with more clients, new clients can be compared in depth to previous ones. Further, the utility of what and how these comparisons are made is evaluated and shaped over time.

Third, there is a great deal of information on how to apply the actual intervention since the therapist has already done it and observed it first hand. The effects of the interventions are interpreted within the entire context of the therapy, including client characteristics, the nature of the therapeutic relationship at that point, the base rates and trends for various client behaviors, and the history of previous interventions with the client.

Fourth, discoveries are made. Because the therapist is immersed in what is going on from moment to moment during the course of therapy, he or she observes the effects of numerous interventions, intended or accidental, and is more likely to make a discovery.

Fifth, threats to internal validity are dealt with. *Internal validity* refers to the ruling out of alternative hypotheses as to why interventions worked. For example, if the therapist offers an interpretation and the client improves over the next few weeks, the internal validity issue concerns the possibility that other factors are responsible for the improvement. Experiments, through the use of a control group, are the easiest way to rule out threats to internal validity, but, as previously discussed, lack relevance (*external validity*). We are not suggesting that therapists say to themselves, "I now will assess systematically the internal validity of my intervention by ruling out rival hypotheses." But, depending on training and background, therapists will consider other factors that could have produced the effect. These factors might include what is going on in the client's life at the time (e.g., the client finally found a job) and the delayed effects of previous interventions. The therapist will then draw upon the wealth of available information and perhaps even ask the client for his or her opinion as to why the improvement occurred. Putting all this together, the therapist decides, with varying degrees of subjective confidence, as to whether or not the interpretation and/or other factors caused the improvement.

Of course, the problem of self-serving bias could influence the process. Many therapists would take such biases into account. For better or worse, therapists do trust their own observations, and data falsification is not a problem. Each clinician assesses threats to internal validity to a level that satisfies his or her own particular criteria. In any event, these personal criteria are no more or no less stringent when applied to evaluating the data presentations (including traditional research studies) of others. All these factors, we believe, contribute to the power that personal experience has in influencing practice.

The idea that internal validity can be assessed without doing an experiment was discussed by Kazdin (1981) in a paper on the methodology of case studies. According to Kazdin, the case study "has had tremendous impact on psychotherapy" (p. 184). Thus, case studies have accomplished the stated purpose of clinical research. Among influential historical cases are Little Hans, Anna O., and Little Albert. Based largely on Kazdin's paper, we have discerned a number of dimensions that characterize influential case studies. These dimensions have much in common with the characteristics that make personal experience influential:

1. *Assessment occasions.* The greater the number of assessment occasions, the easier it is to draw a valid inference (personal experience involves an exceptionally large number of these occasions).

2. *Past and future projections.* Continuous assessment allows for the evaluation of trends and base rates, which, in turn, allows for projecting what would happen in the future without an intervention. An intervention appears effective to the extent that behavior deviates from these future projections. Future projections also can be based on descriptions of a client's problems, history, and daily life. For example, a complete account of a client's relationship history that consistently details characteristics of severe borderline personality disorder would allow one to project that these patterns will persist into the future. If these longstanding patterns change after intervention, confidence is increased that the intervention was responsible for the improvement.

3. *The immediacy and size of effect.* The more immediate and larger an effect, the easier it is to attribute that effect to a particular intervention. The moment-by-moment observation and sensitivity to base rates and

change that personal experience provides would lead to the detection of larger and more immediate effects.

4. *The type of data.* The closer the data are to raw observation, the more influential they are to the audience. Often, such descriptions as transcribed or quoted material are included in case studies. These are close to the raw data accessed in personal experience.

5. *Client descriptions.* In addition to enhancing future projection, detailed information about the client enables practicing clinicians to compare case study subjects to the clients they know. Then the relevance of the case study as well as its credibility can be evaluated.

6. *Intervention description and context.* Case studies are more influential when they include descriptions of what was done, the effects of previous interventions, the conditions leading to the timing of the intervention, and the give-and-take interaction that it produced.

7. *Novelty.* Needless to say, cases are more important when something new is presented.

8. *Assessment of threats to internal validity.* Such assessments can be accomplished in a variety of ways. The reputation of the author could be relevant. For example, if the author is known for critical thinking, openness and awareness about self-serving biases, and sensitivity to internal validity issues, the case is more influential. The details of the case, including attention given to rival hypotheses, are another way to address internal validity.

Intensive local observation, proposed by Cronbach (1975), was suggested by Barlow (1981) as an alternative to traditional research strategies. This method has obvious features in common with both personal experience and influential case studies. Of intensive local observation Cronbach said:

> An observer collecting data in one particular situation is in a position to appraise a practice or proposition in that setting, observing effects in context. In trying to describe and account for what happened, he will give attention to whatever variables were controlled. But he will give equal attention to uncontrolled conditions, to personal characteristics, and to events that occurred during treatment and measurement. As he goes from situation to situation, his first task is to describe and interpret the effect anew in each locale, perhaps taking into account factors unique to that locale. . . . As the results accumulate, a person who seeks understanding will do his best to trace how the uncontrolled factors could have caused the local departures from the mo-

dal effect. That is, generalization comes late and the exception is taken as
seriously as the rule. (pp. 124-125)

Returning now to data collection on FAP, the purpose of research
at this point would be to influence clinical practice. Our therapeutic system must be further developed so that additional guidance can be given
to therapists to detect and appropriately reinforce CRB. Thus, we would
call for data that have characteristics that emulate personal experience,
such as those found in influential case studies and in intensive local observation. These data would have descriptions of what actually happened
in the therapeutic interaction and as much contextual information as possible. The presentation of transcribed material is close to the raw data
and gives the consumer a sense of what actually happened, and whether
the researcher's conclusions are reasonable. The use of videotapes or audiotapes during treatment greatly facilitates this process.

In this book, we have made some small attempts in that direction
by presenting transcribed material to illustrate procedures or phenomena. A more complete presentation would have included transcribed material that (1) was sampled over the course of treatment so that changes
over time could be assessed; (2) formed the basis of the outcome assessment; and (3) entered into the assessment of internal validity. Currently,
studies of this type are under way.

CULTURAL PROBLEMS DUE TO LOSS OF CONTACT

The importance of contact is the central theme of FAP. The more a
client is in touch with the stimuli present in the therapeutic relationship
that evoke CRB, the more she or he will improve. A lack of contact
occurs because of the avoidance of aversiveness. Thus, there is an initial
increase in aversiveness as contact occurs, but over time it is reduced
as positive reinforcement increases.

The theme of increasing contact has thus far been limited to psychotherapy. Yet psychotherapy is a western cultural pursuit mainly available to those who are fortunate enough not to be struggling with meeting
the basic needs of food and shelter. As we sit in our offices doing FAP,
it seems that simply helping individuals lead happier, more productive
lives is not enough in a world that must face poverty, crime, starvation,
drug addiction, pollution, environmental devastation, ozone layer de-
pletion, and the possibility of nuclear annihilation. It is a time when
both therapist and client need to devote more effort to searching for
ways to address these major problems. Perhaps a more socially conscious

psychotherapy could extend the theme of contact beyond interpersonal issues and could focus on how the avoidance of deeper or more hidden contingencies operating in the culture affects societal problems.

In a television show on spiritual life in India, the narrator of the program, an American, was standing on a street in a holy city amid a crowd of people who obviously had little material wealth. He said that Westerners who look at the people in this culture consider them backward and anachronistic. He then mused, perhaps it is us, in the West, who are backward, because we have lost touch with that which is deep inside of us.

We agree that those of us in Western culture may have lost touch, but not with what is deep inside of us. What we have lost touch with is that which is outside of us. This loss of contact has directly contributed to some of the formidable problems that were listed above. Further, we think that at least some of the features of a less materialistic, more spiritually inclined lifestyle can increase contact, and perhaps lead to some solutions to our world's problems.

To illustrate our thoughts on this topic, we would like to examine the Western custom of eating meat. But before doing so, we should point out that the very mention of this topic may evoke strong negative reactions in some of our readers. At least for some people, this negative reaction will result in an inclination to avoid, or an outright avoidance, of our discussion. Our choice of eating the flesh of dead animals as a topic of discussion may illustrate experientially for some readers the concept of avoidance of contact. Incidentally, we are not advocating a position for or against eating meat. We are simply discussing the topic to illustrate how our society helps its citizens to avoid contact in ways that may actually work to our disadvantage.

When we order a fast-food hamburger, it is served in a plastic box and we procure it with money. It tastes good, and we are reinforced for buying and eating it. We have lost touch, however, with the deeper or more hidden contingencies. Our culture has helped us to avoid the fact that the hamburger came from the carcass of an animal that was once alive. It is understandable why this has happened. The division of labor is efficient, practical, and has made our lives more pleasurable. It would be impossible, for example, for one man to raise and to slaughter the cow he eats, to build the Sony Walkman he wants, and to remove his gall bladder when needed.

If we had more contact with the whole process, however, from the birth of the animal to viewing the horrendous conditions under which it lived and died, perhaps we would not eat meat. Alternatively, we might take time to be assured that the animals we ate had a life free of misery and disease and were slaughtered in humane ways.

In his compelling book, *Diet for a New America*, Robbins (1987) explored the less obvious, more remote effects of our high consumption of meat. To mention a few, high meat intake has been linked to heart and circulatory problems. Furthermore, the amount of grain used to produce one meal of meat could be used to make ten meals. The energy and water used in meat production are depleting our natural resources and are contributing to pollution. Rain forests are being cut down to make grazing land for cattle with dire effects on the environment. Thus, less meat eating might improve our health, decrease world hunger, and improve our global environment. These more remote contingencies, however, are almost impossible to contact directly and thus are not likely to have strong motivating effects for most people. These factors might play a larger reinforcing role, however, if there were more contact with the meat-production process. Firsthand experience with feeding the animals, for example, might make more meaningful the argument about the excessive amount of grain that is used.

The point of our illustration is that our culture isolates us from the meat-production process and thereby removes the possible beneficial effects these contingencies could have. We are similarly estranged from other deeper contingencies. For example, we are shielded from the homeless and the hungry, the elderly in nursing homes, people dying, the obtaining of drinking water, the cutting of trees to make paper, and garbage and sewage disposal. Better contact with these processes, although aversive at first, might also improve our lives and have long-term benefits for the planet. The only way to know if the potential benefits would offset the costs, is to somehow increase contact and discover what happens.

Some of the features of a nonmaterialistic and spiritual life seem related to our analysis. We will narrowly define this lifestyle as one in which wealth is not accumulated, the objects one possesses are only those of basic necessity, and the food and clothing required are, as much as possible, made by oneself. An important aspect of the lifestyle is the minimal use of money. As described by Skinner (1986), money is an indirect root of the evil of separating people from the consequences of what they do. Money becomes reinforcing only when it is exchanged for goods and services, and thus "it is always one step away from the from the kind of reinforcing consequences to which the species originally became susceptible" (p. 569).

Another feature of the nonmaterialistic lifestyle is an absence of labor-saving devices. These devices have made Westerners a society of button pushers. We push a button to wash our clothes, to call someone on the phone, and to boil a cup of water. These buttons free us from the aversiveness of the labor that these activities would otherwise require, but insulate us from the deeper contingencies. Thus, the nonmaterialistic lifestyle, along with the minimal use of money and labor-saving devices, would certainly help to bring a person in contact with food production, waste disposal, energy consumption, and the like.

Meditation and prayer are also found in this lifestyle. Although these activities can be viewed as a turning inward, we suggest that in at least some ways they may increase contact with deeper, external contingencies. For example, the act of meditation is inconsistent with many of society's standard rules that separate us from deeper contingencies. Meditation runs counter to such rules as "Always work hard," "Be successful," "Earn lots of money," and "Don't waste time." The activity itself might be conceptualized as practicing the rejection of rules. Rules are the essential fabric of Western society that allows us to learn through the experience of others. Our educational system is based on the dissemination of rules. As Skinner pointed out, however, a drawback of so much of our behavior being rule-governed is that much of what we do is done because we have been told to do it. The deeper reinforcers can be less available. Thus, a meditator breaks the control of rules which might put her or him in a position to contact other reinforcers. Also, meditation might bring more focus on such bodily processes as digestion and heart and circulatory functions, which, in turn, might put the meditator in better contact with those external contingencies that affect these functions.

In this brief discussion, we have looked at how increasing contact with deeper contingencies might be of benefit. It is important to note that the behavior of increasing contact leads not only to more awareness of pain and suffering in the world, but also to an increased awareness of that which is exquisite and sublime. We concur with the viewpoint of Skinner (1986) that the lack of contact with controlling variables causes people in our culture to be "bored, listless, or depressed" (p. 568). We are not, by any means, suggesting that everyone should return to a simple and spiritual life. But perhaps some variation in our present lifestyle which increases contact would not only help us be better psychotherapists, but could enrich our lives in general, and lead us to the exploration of solutions to the more global problems.

CONCLUSION

This book is our interpretation of the psychotherapeutic process. It is based on radical behaviorism and on our behavior that has been contingency-shaped by our clients. Like any interpretation, its value will be measured by its usefulness. If this book produces just one meaningful, intense, client-therapist relationship that otherwise would have not occurred, then, for us, it was useful.

References

Alexander, F., & French, T. M. (1946). *Psychoanalytic therapy: Principles and application.* Lincoln: University of Nebraska Press.

American Psychiatric Association (1987). *Diagnostic and statistical manual of mental disorders* (3rd ed., rev.). Washington, DC: Author.

American Psychological Association (1981). *The ethical principles of psychologists.* Washington, DC: Author.

Barlow, D. H. (1981). On the relation of clinical research to clinical practice. *Journal of Consulting and Clinical Psychology, 49,* 147-155.

Beck, A. T. (1976). *Cognitive therapy and the emotional disorders.* New York: International Universities Press.

Beck, A. T. (1984). Cognition and therapy. *Archives of General Psychiatry, 41,* 1112-1114.

Beck, A. T., Rush, A., Shaw, B., & Emery, G. (1979). *Cognitive therapy of depression.* New York: Guilford Press.

Beck, A. T., Emery, G., & Greenberg, R. L. (1986). *Anxiety disorders and phobias: A cognitive perspective.* New York: Basic Books.

Beidel, B., & Turner, S. (1986). A critique of the theoretical bases of cognitive behavioral theories and therapy. *Clinical Psychology Review, 6,* 177-197.

Bergin, A. S., & Strupp, H. (1972) *Changing frontiers in the science of psychotherapy.* Chicago: Aldine-Atherton.

Cashdan, S. (1988). *Object relations therapy.* New York: Norton.

Catania, A. C. (1984). *Learning.* Englewood Cliffs, NJ: Prentice-Hall.

Chomsky, N. (1959). Review of Skinner's *Verbal Behavior. Language, 35,* 26-58.

Cronbach, L. J. (1975). Beyond the two disciplines of scientific psychology. *American Psychologist, 30,* 116-127.

Day, W. F. (1969). Radical behaviorism in reconciliation with phenomenology. *Journal of the Experimental Analysis of Behavior, 12,* 315-328.

Deci, E. L. (1971). Effects of externally mediated rewards on intrinsic motivation. *Journal of Personality and Social Psychology, 55,* 467-517.

Deikman, A. J. (1973) The meaning of everything. In R. E. Ornstein (Ed.), *The nature of human consciousness.* San Francisco: Freeman.

Diven, K. (1936). Certain determinants in the conditioning of anxiety reactions. *Journal of Psychology, 3,* 291-298.

Dore, J. (1985) Holophrases revisited: Their "logical" development from dialogue. In M. Barret (Ed.), *Children's single word speech*. New York: Wiley.

Eagle, M. N. (1984). *Recent developments in psychoanalysis*. New York: McGraw-Hill.

Efran, J. S., Lukens, R. J., & Lukens, M. D. (1988). Constructivism: What's in it for you? *The Family Therapy Networker, 12*(5), 27-35.

Ellis, A. (1962). *Reason and emotion in psychotherapy*. New York: Lyle Stuart.

Ellis, A. (1970). *The essence of rational emotive therapy: A comprehensive approach to treatment*. New York: Institute for Rational Living.

Erikson, E. (1968). *Identity, youth, and crisis*. New York: Norton.

Ferster, C. B. (1967). Arbitrary and natural reinforcement. *The Psychological Record, 22,* 1-16.

Ferster, C. B. (1972a). Clinical reinforcement. *Seminars in Psychiatry, 4*(2), 101-111.

Ferster, C. B. (1972b). An experimental analysis of clinical phenomena. *The Psychological Record, 22,* 1-16.

Ferster, C. B. (1972c). Psychotherapy from the standpoint of a behaviorist. In J. D. Keehn (Ed.), *Psychopathology in animals: Research and clinical implications*. New York: Academic Press.

Ferster, C. B. (1979). A laboratory model of psychotherapy. In P. Sjoden (Ed.), *Trends in behavior therapy*. New York: Academic Press.

Freud, S. (1958). The dynamics of transference. In J. Strachey (Ed. and Trans.), *The standard edition of the complete psychological works of Sigmund Freud* (Vol. 12, pp. 99-108). London: Hogarth Press. (Original work published 1912)

Freud, S. (1959). An autobiographical study. In J. Strachey (Ed. and Trans.), *The standard edition of the complete psychological works of Sigmund Freud* (Vol. 20, pp. 19-71). London: Hogarth Press. (Original work published 1925)

Furman, B., & Ahola, T. (1988) Seven illusions. *The Family Therapy Networker, 12*(5), 30-31.

Gill, M. M., & Hoffman, I. Z. (1982). A method for studying the analysis of aspects of the patient's experience of the relationship in psychoanalysis and psychotherapy. *Journal of the American Psychoanalytic Association, 30,* 137-167.

Goldfried, M. R., & Davison, G. C. (1976). *Clinical behavior therapy*. New York: Holt, Rinehart & Winston.

Goldfried, M. R.(1982). Resistance and clinical behavior therapy. In P. L. Wachtel (Ed.), *Resistance: Psychodynamic and behavioral approaches* (pp. 95-113). New York: Plenum Press.

Greben, S. E. (1981). The essence of psychotherapy. *British Journal of Psychiatry, 138,* 449-455.

Greenacre, P. (1954). The role of transference. Practical considerations in relation to psychoanalytic psychotherapy. *Journal of the American Psychoanalytical Association, 2,* 671-684

Greenberg, L. S., & Pinsof, W. M. (1986). *The psycotherapeutic process: A research handbook*. New York: Guilford Press

Greenson, R. R. (1972). Beyond transference and interpretation. *International Journal of Psychoanalysis, 53,* 213-217.

Greenwald, A. E. (1982). Is anyone in charge? Personalysis versus the principle of personal unity. In J. Suls (Ed.), *Psychological perspectives on the self* (Vol. 1, pp 151-181). Hillsdale, NJ: Erlbaum.

Guidano, V. F., & Liotti, G. (1983). *Cognitive processes and emotional disorders*. New York: Guilford Press.

Hawkins, R. P., & Dobes, R. W. (1977). Behavioral definitions in applied behavior analysis: Explicit or implicit? In B. C. Etzel, J. M. LeBlanc, & D. M. Baer (Eds.), *New developments in behavioral research*. Hillsdale, NJ: Erlbaum.

Hayes, S. C. (1984). Making sense of spirituality. *Behaviorism, 12,* 99-110.

Hayes, S. C. (1987). A contextual approach to therapeutic change. In N. S. Jacobson (Ed.), *Psychotherapists in clinical practice: Cognitive and behavioral perspectives* (pp. 327-387). New York: Guilford Press.

Hollon, S. D., & Kriss, M. R. (1984). Cognitive factors in clinical research and practice. *Clinical Psychology Review, 4*, 35-76.

Jacobson, N. S. (1989). The therapist-client relationship in cognitive behavior therapy: Implications for treating depression. *Journal of Cognitive Psychotherapy, 3*, 85-96.

Kazdin, A. E. (1975). *Behavior modification in applied settings.* Chicago: Dorsey Press.

Kazdin, A. E. (1981). Drawing valid inferences from case studies. *Journal of Consulting and Clinical Psychology, 49*, 183-192.

Kernberg, O. (1976). *Object relations theory and clinical psychoanalysis.* New York: Jason Aronson.

Keith-Spiegel, P., & Koocher, G. P. (1985). *Ethics in psychology: Professional standards and cases.* New York: Random House.

Klein, D. F. (1974). Endogenomorphic depression. *Archives of General Psychiatry, 31*, 447-454.

Klein, M. (1952). Some theoretical conclusions regarding the emotional life of the infant. In M. Klein (Ed.), *Envy, gratitude and other works, 1946-1963.* New York: Delacorte Press.

Kohlenberg, R. J. (1973). Operant control of multiple personality. *Behavior Therapy, 4*, 137-140.

Kohlenberg, R. J., & Tsai, M. (1987). Functional analytic psychotherapy. In N. S. Jacobson (Ed.), *Psychotherapists in clinical practice: Cognitive and behavioral perspectives* (pp. 388-443). New York: Guilford Press.

Kohut, H. (1971). *The analysis of the self.* New York: International Universities Press.

Kohut, H. (1977). *The restoration of the self.* New York: International Universities Press.

Krantz, S. E. (1985). When depressive cognitions reflect negative realities. *Cognitive Therapy and Research, 9* (6), 595-610.

Langs, R. (1976). *The therapeutic interaction, Vol. II.* New York: Jason Aronson.

Langs, R. (1982). Countertransference. In S. R. Slipp (Ed.), *Curative factors in dynamic psychotherapy* (pp. 127-152). New York: McGraw-Hill.

Levine, F. M., & Fasnacht, G. (1974). Token rewards may lead to token learning. *American Psychologist, 29*, 816-820.

Linehan, M. M. (1987). Dialectical behavior therapy for borderline personality disorder: Theory and method. *Bulletin of the Menninger Clinic, 51*, 261-276.

Lutzker, J. R., & Martin, J. A. (1981). *Behavior change.* Monterey, CA: Brooks/Cole.

Mahler, M.(1952). On child psychosis and schizophrenia: Autistic and symbiotic infantile psychoses. *Psychoanalytic Study of the Child, 7*, 206-305.

Mahrer, A. R. (1988). Discovery-oriented psychotherapy research. *American Psychologist, 43*, 694-702.

Marziali, E. A. (1984). Prediction of outcome of brief psychotherapy from therapist interpretive interventions. *Archives of General Psychiatry, 41*, 310-304.

Masson, J. M. (1988). *Against therapy.* New York: Atheneum.

Masterson, J. F. (1985). *The real self.* New York: Brunner/Mazel.

Messer, S. B. (1983). Integrating psychoanalytic and behavior therapy: Limitations, possibilities and trade-offs. *British Journal of Clinical Psychology, 22*, 131-132.

Messer, S. B. (1986). Behavioral and psychoanalytic perspectives at therapeutic choice points. *American Psychologist, 41*(11), 1261-1272.

Miller, A. K. (1983). *The dramas of the gifted child.* New York: Basic Books.

Nichols, M.P., & Efran, J. (1985). Catharsis in psychotherapy: a new perspective. *Psychotherapy: Theory, Research and Practice, 22*(1), 46-58.

Paolino, T. J., Jr. (1981). *Psychoanalytic psychotherapy.* New York: Brunner/Mazel.

Peck, M. S. (1978). *The road less traveled*. New York: Simon & Schuster.

Peck, M. S. (1987). *The different drum: Community-making and peace*. New York: Simon and Schuster.

Putnam, F. W. (1989). *Diagnosis and treatment of multiple personality disorder*. New York: Guilford Press.

Quattrone, G. A. (1985). On the congruity between internal states and action. *Psychological Bulletin, 98*, 3-30.

Reese, E. P. (1966). *The analysis of human operant behavior*. Dubuque, IA: Wm. C. Brown.

Rice, L. N., & Greenberg, L. S. (1984). *Patterns of change*. New York: Guilford Press.

Robbins, J. (1987). *Diet for a new America*. Walpole, NH: Stillpoint Publishing.

Rogers, C. R. (1961). *On becoming a person*. Boston: Houghton Mifflin.

Russell, P. L., & Brandsma, J. M. (1974). A theoretical and empirical integration of the rational emotive and classical conditioning theories. *Journal of Consulting and Clinical Psychology, 42*(3), 389-397.

Safran, J. D., Vallis, T. M., Segal, Z. V., & Shaw, B. F., (1986). Assessment of core cognitive processes in cognitive therapy. *Cognitive Therapy and Research, 10* (5), 509-526.

Scott, R., Himadi, W., & Keane, T. (1983). Generalization of social skills. In M. Hersen, R. Eisler, & P. Miller (Eds.), *Progress in behavior modification*. New York: Academic Press.

Searles, H. (1959). The effort to drive the other person crazy: An element in the aetiology and treatment of schizophrenia. *British Journal of Medical Psychology, 32*, 1-18.

Silverman, J., Silverman, J. D., & Eardley, D. (1984). In reply. *Archives of General Psychiatry, 41*, 1112.

Sizemore, C. C. (1989). *A mind of my own*. New York: William Morrow.

Skinner, B. F. (1953). *Science and human behavior*. New York: Macmillan.

Skinner, B. F. (1957). *Verbal behavior*. New York: Appleton-Century-Crofts.

Skinner, B. F. (1969). *Contingencies of reinforcement*. New York: Appleton-Century-Crofts.

Skinner, B. F. (1971). *Beyond freedom and dignity*. New York: Knopf.

Skinner, B. F. (1974). *About behaviorism*. New York: Knopf.

Skinner, B. F. (1986). What is wrong with daily life in the western world. *American Psychologist, 41*, 568-574

Skinner, B. F. (1989). *Recent issues in the analysis of behavior*. Columbus, OH: Merrill.

Sterba, R. F. (1934). The fate of the ego in psychoanalysis. *International Journal of Psycho-Analysis, 15*, 117-126.

Stone, M. H. (1982). Turning points in psychotherapy. In S. R. Slipp (Ed.), *Curative factors in dynamic psychotherapy* (pp. 259-279). New York: McGraw-Hill.

Sweet, A. A. (1984). The therapeutic relationship in behavior therapy. *Clinical Psychology Review, 4*, 253-272.

Truax, C. B. (1966). Reinforcement and nonreinforcement in Rogerian psychotherapy. *Journal of Abnormal Psychology, 21*(1), 1-9.

Turk, D., & Salovey, P. (1985). Cognitive structures, processes and cognitive behavior modification. *Cognitive Therapy and Research, 9*, 1-17.

Wachtel, P. L. (1977). *Psychoanalysis and behavior therapy: Toward an integration*. New York: Basic Books.

Waterhouse, G., & Strupp, H. (1984). The patient therapist relationship: Research from the psychodynamic perspective. *Clinical Psychology Review, 4*, 77-92.

Wessells, M. G. (1982). A critique on Skinner's views of the obstructive character of cognitive theories. *Behaviorism, 10*, 65- 84.

Winnicott, D. W. (1965) *The family and individual development*. New York: Basic Books.

Woolfolk, R. L., & Messer, S. B. (1988). Introduction to hermeneutics. In S. B. Messer, L. A. Sass & R. L. Woolfolk (Eds.), *Hermeneutics and psychological theory* (pp. 2-26). New Brunswick, NJ: Rutgers University Press.

Zettle, R. D. (1980). *Insight: Rules and revelations.* Paper presented at the meeting of the The Association for the Advancement of Behavior Therapy, New York.

Zettle, R. D., & Hayes, S. C. (1982). Rule governed behavior: A potential theoretical framework for cognitive-behavioral therapy. In P. C. Kendall (Ed.), *Advances in cognitive behavioral research and therapy* (Vol. 1). New York: Academic Press.

Zuriff, G. (1987). Naturalistic ethics. In S. Modigil & C. Modgil (Eds.), *B. F. Skinner: Consensus and controversy* (pp. 309-318). New York: Falmer Press.

Index

Ahola, T., 5
Alexander, F., 172, 173
Amnesia, 83
American Psychological Association
    (APA), 189
Applied behavior analysis, 7, 8, 10
Assertiveness, 20, 25, 78, 104
Assessment, 23
Aversive stimuli, 32-33, 77-78, 89-92

Barlow, D.H., 198, 199, 202
Beck, A.T., 98, 99, 101, 102, 115, 116, 121
Behavior therapy, and FAP, 182-185
Beidel, B., 100
Bergin, A.S., 199
Borderline personality disorder, 149-151
Brandsma, J.M., 98

Cashdan, S., 180, 181
Catania, A.C., 82, 141
Clinically relevant behavior, 13-14, 17-18
Cognition, 101-103
    structures, 113-114
    see also Thought-behavior relationship
Contingency, see Reinforcement
Cronbach, L.J., 202
Cognitive therapy, 98-103
Contact, 7, 37, 38
    and cultural problems, 203-206
    during therapy, 78-81
Contextualism, 4
Controlling variables, 5
Conventional behaviorism, 2
CRB1, 18-19

CRB2, 19-22
CRB3, 23

Davison, G.C., 183
Day, W.F., 6
Deci, E.L., 12
Deikman, A.J., 126, 140, 141
Discriminative function, 17-18
Discriminative stimulus (Sd), 17, 38-39,
    54-55
Disguised mand, 57-58
Diven, K., 171
Dobes, R.W., 14
Dore, J., 132
DSM-III-R, 2, 30

Eagle, M.N., 179
Eardley, D., 100
Efran, J.S., 3, 4
Eliciting function, 17-18
Ellis, A., 98, 106
Emery, G., 98, 102
Erikson, E., 126
Ethics, 189-194
    defined behaviorally, 189-191
Experience, behavioral account of, 127-128

Fasnacht, G., 12
Feelings
    avoidance of, 77-78, 85, 92
    definition, 69
    expressing, 65-66, 75-76
    importance in therapy, 78-81, 86-87

Feelings (cont.)
  learning about, 72-73, 155-156
  therapist's expression of, 31, 34, 66,
    87-88, 95-96
  what is felt, 70
Ferster, C.B., 10, 29, 32, 38
Forgetting, 83
Formal analysis, 57
Free association, 28, 159-165
French, T.M., 172, 173
Freud, S., 170, 171, 175, 176, 177
Functional analysis, 6, 15, 57
Functional relationship, 6, 38-40
Functional units
  size of, 130-132
  of· verbal behavior, 130-131
Furman, B., 5

Generalization, 15, 171
Gill, M.M., 174
Goldfried, M.R., 183
Greben, S., 1, 27
Greenacre, P., 175
Greenberg, L.S., 199
Greenberg, R.L., 102
Greenson, R.R., 174
Greenwald, A.E., 125
Guidano, V.F., 98, 102

Hawkins, R.P., 14
Hayes, S.C., 4, 7, 24, 37, 74, 111, 139
Headache, 90
Himadi, W., 184
Hoffman, I.Z., 174
Hollon, S.D., 98, 100, 101, 102, 114
Homework assignments, 28
Hypnosis, 28, 154-155

Identity, see Self
Imagery exercises, 28
Interpretation, 37-38
  and feelings, 85
  and thought-behavior relationship,
    119-120, 123
Intimacy, 10, 27, 31, 75, 143
Intraverbal, 53-54, 56-57

Jacobson, N.S., 113, 114, 116

Kazdin, A.E., 7, 201
Keane, T., 184
Kernberg, O., 179

Kieth-Spiegel, P., 189, 190
Klein, D.F., 99
Klein, M., 179
Kohlenberg, R.J., 7, 153
Kohut, H., 147, 179
Koocher, G.P., 189, 190
Krantz, S.E., 100
Kriss, M.R., 98, 100, 101, 102, 114

Langs, R., 172, 173, 175
Levine, F.M., 12
Linehan, M.M., 149
Liotti, G., 98, 102
Lukens, M.D., 3
Lukens, R.J., 3
Lutzker, J.R., 7

Mahler, M., 179
Mahrer, A.R., 199
Mand, 52-54, 56, 105-111
  disguised, 57-58
Martin, J.A., 7
Marziali, E.A., 26
Masson, J.M., 193
Masterson, J.F., 126
Matarazzo, J., 199
Meaning, of verbal Behavior, 58
Mentalism, 5
Messer, S.B., 37, 188
Metaphors, 52, 59
Methodological behaviorism, 2
Miller, A.K., 147
Multiple causation, 58-59
Multiple personality disorder, 151-157

Narcissistic personality disorder, 147-148

Operant behavior, 17, 71, 79

Paolino, T.J., Jr., 177, 178
Passivity, of therapist, 27, 158-159
Peck, M.S., 3, 27, 32
Perspective, 139
Pinsoff, W.M., 199
Psychoanalysis, 37, 49, 60
  and FAP, 170-182, 185-188
Punishment, see Aversive stimuli
Putnam, F.W., 151, 154, 156, 157

Quattrone, G.A., 100

Racism, 192

Radical behaviorism, 1, 2, 3-8
Reese, E.P., 7
Reinforcement, 8-10, 36-37, 104
    arbitrary and natural, 10-13, 29-35
    and cognitive structures, 113-114
Reinforcing function, 17-18
Remembering, 4, 5, 19-20, 81-84
Repression, see Remembering
Research, pitfalls of, 197-199
    alternative methods, 198-203
    discovery and, 199, 200
Respondent behavior, 17, 70-71, 79, 82
Response selection, 59
Rice, L.N., 199
Robbins, J., 205
Rogers, C.R., 31, 169
Rules, 111-113
    examples of, 164
    and psychoanalysis, 175
Rush, A., 98
Russell, P.L., 98

Safran, J.D., 101
Salovey, P., 98
Scott, R., 184
Sd (discriminative stimulus), 17, 38-39,
    54-55
Segal, Z.V., 101
Self
    behavioral account of, 128-139
    definitions of, 126-127
    observation, 22, 60
    problems of, 141-157
Self-disclosure, see Feelings, Therapist
Sensitivity, 47
Sensitivity to criticism, 91-92, 145-146, 147
Sexism, 192
Shaw, B., 98
Shaw, B.F., 101
Silverman, J., 100
Silverman, J.D., 100
Sizemore, C.C., 156, 157
Skinner, B.F., 1, 2, 3, 5, 6, 7, 8, 24, 47, 49,
    50, 52, 54, 57, 59, 69, 70, 106, 108,
    111, 112, 127, 130, 131, 134, 146, 189,
    205, 206

Social Skills Training, 78
Sr (reinforcer), 38-39
Sterba, R.F., 178
Stimulus control, 129, see also Sd
Stimulus functions, 17
Stone, M.H., 175
Strupp, H., 175, 199
Subtle responses, 60
Supervision, 195-196
Supplementary stimulation, 58-59
Sweet, A.A., 183

Tact, 52-56, 72, 105-111, 129-130
Therapeutic alliance, 177-179
Therapeutic relationship, 26-27, 169-170,
    193-191, 195
Thinking, definition of, 106
Thought-behavior relationship, 97-113
Transference, 26, 170-177
Trauma
    and MPD, 151-157
    and remembering, 83
Truax, C.B., 31
Trust, 20-21, 28-29
Tsai, M., 7
Turk, D., 98
Turner, S., 100

Unconscious, 9, 104, 113
    meaning, 47-50, 58-59, 60

Validity, 200
Vallis, T.M., 101
Verbal behavior, meaning of, 58
Vulnerability, 77

Wachtel, P.L., 29
Waterhouse, G., 175
Wessells, M.G., 114
Western culture, 204
Winnicott, D.W., 126
Woolfolk, R.L., 37

Zettle, R.D., 24, 37, 83, 111
Zuriff, G., 189

Printed in the United States
71475LV00002B/328-339

9 780306 438578